The Fat, Fibre and Carbohydrate Counter

The essential guide to healthy eating

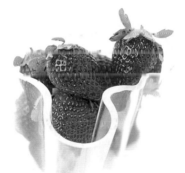

Select Editions, Vancouver

First published in Canada in 2002 by
Select Editions
8036 Enterprise Street
Burnaby, British Columbia
V5A 1V7 Canada
Tel: (604) 415-2444
Fax: (604) 415-3444

Consultant Editor: Dell Stanford
Nutritional data provided by: Jenny Copeland
Project Editors: Angela Newton and Anna Nicholas
Concept and Design: Marylouise Brammer
UK Design: Cathy Layzell and Fay Singer

CEO: Robert Oerton
Publisher: Catie Ziller
Production Manager: Lucy Byrne

Illustrations by Lorraine Harrison
Photography by Ben Deamley

Colour separation by Colourscan in Singapore
Printed in Hong Kong by Wing King Tong

ISBN 1 85391 803 2
© Text, design and photography Murdoch Books UK 1999
© Illustrations Murdoch Books UK 1999
The Food Wheel p6: based on The Balance of Good Health, courtesy of the
Health Education Authority.

Murdoch Books is a trademark of Murdoch Magazines Pty Ltd.
A catalogue record for this book is available from the British Library.

NUTRITION: The nutritional values are approximations and can be affected by biological
and seasonal variations in foods, the unknown composition of some manufactured foods
nd uncertainty in the dietary database. All figures have been checked, and where necessary
recalculated, using McCance & Widdowson's composition of foods – 5th edition (MAFF) and
its supplements. Fibre values have been calculated using the Englyst method.

IMPORTANT: This book is intended solely as a guide for following a healthy diet. Anybody
with specific dietary needs, or the elderly, pregnant women, young children and those suffering
from immune deficiency diseases should consult their GP before changing their diets.

CONTENTS

Your Fat & Carbohydrate Requirements 4

Finding the Right Balance 6

Vitamins & Minerals 10

Food Terms 12

Nutrition Labelling 16

Food Composition Chart 18

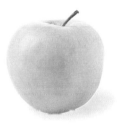

HOW TO USE THIS BOOK

The Fat, Fibre and Carbohydrate Counter provides all the information you need to follow a healthy diet. Use the following few pages to identify your personal dietary needs, to understand the role of food in maintaining good health and to establish just how much nutrition your diet provides. The Vitamins and Minerals Chart, together with the pages on Food Terms and Food Labelling then provide you with all the tools you need to identify what foods you should eat as part of a healthy diet.

The Food Composition Chart contains fibre, carbohydrate and energy values for most commonly available foods. The figure next to each food represents the average serving,

but if the food has no typical serving, as is the case with flour, a 100g amount is given. In the fibre column, N denotes that the figure has not been calculated, + that amounts have been detected but not accurately calculated and Tr means that only a trace (less than 0.1g) has been found.

The right hand pages of the chart focus on particular foods, providing useful information about different varieties, healthy recipe variations and hints and tips for making the foods part of a balanced diet. Essential tips on the best choices for everyday shopping is combined with notes on how to opt for lower-fat versions, and how taste needn't be compromised for health.

YOUR FAT & CARBOHYDRATE REQUIREMENTS

Everyone has different fat and carbohydrate requirements. The amount of calories you should be consuming each day depends on a number of different factors, including your age, sex, weight and activity level.

By following these four straightforward instructions, you can work out how many calories you need to consume every day in order to maintain a healthy and balanced diet. The results are only approximate – even those people who are the same sex, age, weight and activity level will have different energy requirements.

STEP 1

The amount of calories you need each day depends both on your age and how much you weigh. In order to calculate your estimated calorie requirement, place your weight in kilograms in the appropriate equation for your age (see right).

STEP 2

Your body will require more or less calories depending on how active you are, both at work and during your leisure time. Multiply your calorie requirement from Step 1 by your activity level below. For example, if you are a woman and work in an office but do

STEP 1 – FOR MEN	
18–29y	$[(0.063 \times weight) + 2.896] \times 239$
30–60y	$[(0.048 \times weight) + 3.653] \times 239$
Over 60y	$[(0.049 \times weight) + 2.459] \times 239$

STEP 1 – FOR WOMEN	
18–29y	$[(0.062 \times weight) + 2.036] \times 239$
30–60y	$[(0.034 \times weight) + 3.538] \times 239$
Over 60y	$[(0.038 \times weight) + 2.755] \times 239$

some form of exercise on most days, then your occupational activity level is 'light' but your non-occupational activity level will be 'moderately active'. So your overall activity level will be 1.5 (these levels are approximate).

Non-occupational activity	Occupational activity					
	light		moderate		moderate/heavy	
	male	female	male	female	male	female
Non-active	1.4	1.4	1.6	1.5	1.7	1.5
Moderately active	1.5	1.5	1.7	1.6	1.8	1.6
Very active	1.6	1.6	1.8	1.7	1.9	1.7

STEP 3

If you are trying to lose or gain weight, then you will need to reduce or increase the number of calories you consume every day. The best way of doing this is to subtract 500 calories from your estimated daily calorie needs. If you want to increase your weight, then add 500 calories. You have now calculated your average daily calorie needs.

The fact that you only need to reduce your calorie intake by 500 calories per day may come as a surprise to some people. However, this is by far the best way to go about dieting because it will enable you to lose 1lb per week. If you lose weight in a slow and steady manner, then you are much more likely to keep the weight off permanently than if you lose weight very quickly. Crash dieting is not the answer.

STEP 4

You can now calculate how many grams of fat and carbohydrate you should aim to eat each day for good health.

● No more than 35% of the calories you eat each day should come from fats. To calculate what this means in terms of the amount of fat you should be eating, place your calorie requirement into this equation:

$$\frac{(calories/day \times 0.35)}{9} = grams\ fat\ each\ day$$

● At least 50% of the calories you eat each day should come from carbohydrates. To calculate the grams of carbohydrates, place your calorie requirement into this equation:

$$\frac{(calories \times 0.5)}{3.75} = grams\ carbohydrate\ each\ day$$

SAMPLE CALCULATION

Jane is 36 years old, weighs 72kg and is 163cm tall. She has a 'light' occupation activity level and is moderately active out of work. She is trying to lose weight (see the Body Mass Index chart on page 9). Her estimated requirements are:

STEP 1 – Estimated calorie requirement

$[(0.034 \times 72) + 3.538] \times 239 = 1430$ calories / day

STEP 2 – Estimated calorie requirement determined by activity level

$1430 \times 1.5 = 2146$ calories / day

STEP 3 – Recommended caloric requirement to lose weight

$2146 - 500 = 1646$ calories / day

STEP 4 – Recommended fat and carbohydrate allowance per day

Grams of fat each day: $\frac{(1646 \times 0.35)}{9} = 64g$ / day

Grams of carbohydrate each day: $\frac{(1646 \times 0.5)}{3.75} = 219g$ / day

FINDING THE RIGHT BALANCE

Eating a wide variety of different foods in the right proportions and enjoying it is the key to a healthy diet! A combination of regular physical activity and a healthy diet not only helps you to stay in shape, but it also reduces your risk of developing conditions such as heart disease, cancer, constipation and osteoporosis.

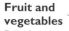

Fruit and vegetables
Full of nutrients, these foods should make up a large portion of your diet.

Bread, other cereals and potatoes
These foods should make up the bulk of your diet because they are low in fat and often high in fibre.

Meat, fish and alternatives
These foods are a good source of protein but are best eaten in moderation.

Milk and dairy products
Eat these in moderation because these foods tend to be high in fat.

Foods containing fat and/or sugar
Limit your intake of these foods because they can lead to obesity or tooth decay.

EATING A BALANCED DIET

There's no such thing as an 'unhealthy' food, only an 'unhealthy' diet . Therefore, eating healthily doesn't necessarily mean cutting out all your favourite foods but eating the right balance does mean eating more of some types of food than others. For example, at least half of the total calories that we eat should come from starchy foods, such as bread, potatoes, pasta and rice, which are high in carbohydrates. Fat should contribute

no more than 35% of the total calories that we eat. It can be difficult to know what this means in practical terms, but with the help of this book, eating healthily and maintaining a healthy weight will become second nature.

The diagram above, the food wheel, represents the recommended balance of foods in the diet, showing how much of each type of food we should aim to eat.

Bread, other cereals and potatoes

At least 50% of the calories we eat should come from the starchy foods included in this group. Because they are bulky, low in fat and often high in fibre, these foods fill us up without providing too many calories. It's what you serve with them (for example, butter on bread) that add the fat and calories. This group also includes breakfast cereals, oats, pasta, noodles, plantains, beans and lentils. These foods provide carbohydrate (starch), some calcium and iron, and B vitamins. Make these foods the main part of most meals.

Fruit and vegetables

Eat plenty of these foods – aim for at least five portions a day (a glass of fruit juice can count as one portion). Choose from a wide variety of fresh, frozen or canned fruits and vegetables. Contrary to popular belief, frozen fruit and vegetables can be just as nutritious as fresh (if not more so) because they are usually frozen immediately after harvesting, reducing nutrient loss. They are full of antioxidant vitamins, especially vitamin C and carotenes (vitamin A), as well as folates, fibre and some carbohydrates. In addition, they are low in fat and calories.

Milk and dairy products

Eat moderate amounts of these foods and choose lower fat alternatives where possible. This group includes milk, cheese, yoghurt and fromage frais, but it doesn't include butter, eggs and cream. Milk and dairy products provide calcium, protein, vitamins B12, A and D. Although semi-skimmed and skimmed milk contain less of the fat soluble vitamins A and D, their calcium content is the same as full-fat milk.

Meat, fish and alternatives

Eat moderate amounts of these foods and choose lower fat alternatives where possible. This group includes eggs, nuts, textured vegetable protein, tofu, beans and lentils. Aim to eat at least two portions of fish per week, one of which should be an oily fish. These foods provide iron, protein, B vitamins, zinc and magnesium.

Foods containing fat and/or sugar

Eat these types of foods sparingly and choose low-fat alternatives where possible. This group includes butter, other fat spreads, oils, salad dressings and treats such as biscuits, cakes, chocolate, ice cream, sweets, crisps and sweetened drinks. Sugary foods should be limited because eating them frequently can lead to tooth decay.

FATS

Small amounts of fat are essential to a healthy diet – they provide fat soluble vitamins A, D, E and K, as well as essential fatty acids.

Eating the right amount of fat

Most of us eat too much fat. Currently fat provides about 40% of the calories eaten. This needs to be reduced to no more than 35%. There are two main reasons why eating too much fat is bad for us:

● Fat contains more calories per gram (9kcal/g) than carbohydrates (3.75kcals/g), protein (4kcals/g) or alcohol (7kcals/g). This means that foods containing a high proportion of fat tend to be high in calories. So, eating them in large amounts is likely to lead to weight gain and obesity.

● Eating too much fat, especially saturated fat, increases the risk that you might develop heart disease.

Eating the right sort of fat

It's not just the total amount of fat we eat that can affect our health, but also the type of fat. Fat is made up of units called fatty acids and there are three main types of fatty acids – saturated, monounsaturated and polyunsaturated. The fat in food contains a mixture of all three types, but different foods contain different proportions of each type.

Saturated fat

Foods that contain a high proportion of saturated fats include some milk and dairy products and meat and meat products. They are also found in palm and coconut oil and some spreading fats, hard cooking fats, biscuits, cakes and pastries. Eating too much saturated fat increases levels of blood cholesterol. Cholesterol is made mostly by the liver and is carried in the blood by proteins called LDL's and HDL's. LDL cholesterol is sometimes referred to as 'bad' cholesterol because high blood levels can result in cholesterol being deposited on the blood vessel walls, eventually leading to atherosclerosis and possibly a heart attack. HDL cholesterol, on the other hand, is often referred to as 'good' cholesterol because it carries the cholesterol to the liver for disposal.

Monounsaturated fats

Monounsaturates are the main type of fat found in olive and rapeseed oils. They are also found in some spreading fats, nuts, avocados, milk and dairy products and meat. When saturates in the diet are replaced by monounsaturated, 'bad' cholesterol levels are reduced and the risk of heart disease lowered.

Polyunsaturated fats

There are two main groups of polyunsaturates known as n-6 and n-3 according to their structure. When saturates in the diet are replaced by n-6 polyunsaturates (found in sunflower, corn and soya bean oils, spreads high in polyunsaturates and meat), levels of 'bad' cholesterol in the blood are reduced. However, it is also likely that 'good' cholesterol levels are also reduced. Current dietary guidelines recommend that we do not increase our intake of polyunsaturates any further and that we should aim to replace the saturates in our diet with monounsaturates as well as polyunsaturates.

n-3 polyunsaturates are the main types of fat found in oily fish such as mackerel, pilchards, sardines, trout and salmon. These fats are sometimes referred to as omega-3 fatty acids and some spreading fats are now enriched with them. These types of fats have no effect on blood cholesterol levels, but they do reduce the tendency of blood to clot, thereby reducing the risk of heart disease.

Trans fatty acids

Trans fatty acids (trans fats) occur naturally in dairy foods such as butter and fat from beef and lamb. They are also produced during margarine manufacture. This process, hydrogenation, produces hydrogenated fats. If hydrogenated fats/oils are included in an ingredients list, this indicates that a food contains trans fats. This fat is often found in spreading fats, biscuits and cakes. Trans fats may have undesirable effects on cholesterol levels (in a similar way to saturated fats) and you should limit the amount you eat.

What about cholesterol intake?

Did you know that the amount of cholesterol we eat has only a very small effect on the amount of cholesterol in our blood? If we eat large quantities of cholesterol, the body responds by producing less, so the overall effect on blood cholesterol levels will be small. Increasing saturated fat intake and becoming obese are the most likely causes of increasing blood cholesterol levels.

FIBRE

Fibre is the non-digestible part of food. It includes two types of fibre; soluble and insoluble. The soluble fibre, which is found in oats, pulses, fruit and vegetables, may help lower blood cholesterol levels if consumed as part of a diet low in saturated fats. The insoluble fibre found in foods such as bread, pasta, rice and cereals reduces constipation and the risk of other bowel disorders.

On average, we eat about 12g of fibre a day. According to healthy eating guidelines, this should be increased to 18g per day. The two food groups 'bread, other cereals and potatoes' and 'fruit and vegetables' illustrated in the food wheel on page 6 are good sources of dietary fibre. Making sure that these foods make up two-thirds of your diet would significantly increase your fibre intake.

Are you a healthy weight?

Health experts use Body Mass Index (BMI) to assess people's weight. You can calculate your own BMI by using the following equation or by simply plotting your weight on the chart below:

weight (kg)/ height² (m) = BMI

eg 72kg/1.63²m − 27 BMI

BMI criteria

Less than 18	Underweight
18–20	OK – a healthy weight but do not lose any more
20–25	OK – a healthy weight
25–30	Overweight
30–40	Fat
Over 40	Very fat

Body Mass Index Chart

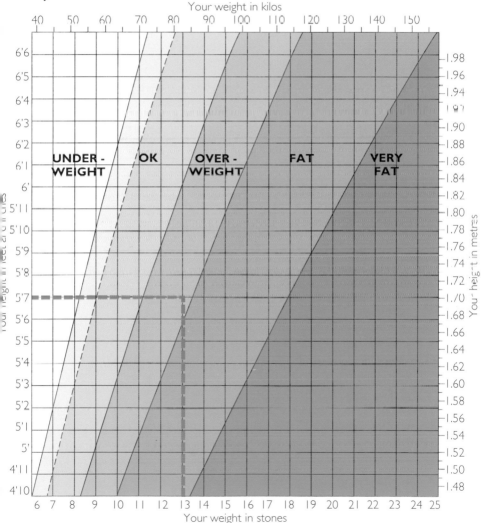

VITAMINS & MINERALS

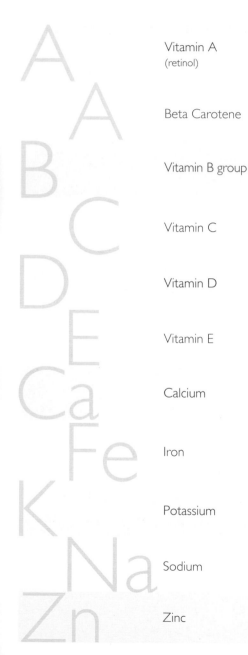

FUNCTIONS

Vitamin A
(retinol)

Maintains healthy vision, skin, teeth and bones as well as many important mucus membranes such as those found in the throat, nose, lungs and intestines. Important for the growth of children.

Beta Carotene

A form of vitamin A converted into retinol in the intestines. It is a powerful antioxidant vitamin (see Food Terms on page 12).

Vitamin B group

These vitamins work together, enabling energy to be released from the food we eat. They are also vital for the production of antibodies, red blood cells, healthy skin and muscle tissue.

Vitamin C

Protects against infection and is required for the production of collagen and connective body tissue. Aids absorption of iron from non-animal sources and helps maintain a healthy body.

Vitamin D

The 'sunshine' vitamin made under the skin when exposed to sunlight. Essential for the proper use of calcium and phosphorous, which are needed for the maintenance of healthy bones.

Vitamin E

An antioxidant vitamin (see Food terms) that is essential for the maintenance of cell membranes.

Calcium

Development and maintenance of healthy bones and teeth. It also has an important role in blood clotting and the regulation of heartbeat.

Iron

Essential for the production of red blood cells that carry oxygen around the body. It also helps the body to fight off infection.

Potassium

Maintains nerves, cells and muscle tissue. Together with sodium, potassium also helps to regulate water balance and blood pressure.

Sodium

Essential for muscle and nerve activity. Works with potassium to control the body's water balance and maintain blood pressure.

Zinc

Needed for normal growth and development of reproductive organs, teeth, bones and the body's defence system. Aids healing and appetite.

DEFICIENCY / EXCESS PROBLEMS	SOURCES

Deficiency can cause eye, skin and hair problems, and an increased susceptibility to infections. Excessive amounts can be toxic and should be avoided by pregnant women.

Liver, kidneys, fish liver oil, eggs, dairy foods, butter and margarine. Vitamin A is fat soluble so reduced fat dairy products contain less vitamin A than full-fat varieties.

Deficiency can lead to an increased susceptibility to infections. Large doses of purified beta carotene supplements have been known to cause the skin to turn an orange colour.

Fruit and vegetables, particularly yellow, green, orange and red varieties such as carrots, tomatoes, spinach, watercress, broccoli, peppers and apricots.

Deficiency can lead to anaemia, fatigue, skin problems and depression. Heavy drinkers, smokers women on contraceptive pills and vegans may need extra vitamin B, as may vegans.

Liver, kidneys, meat, poultry, fish, yeast, wholegrain breads and cereals, seeds, nuts, legumes, eggs, milk, cheese, yogurt and leafy green vegetables.

Deficiency can increase susceptibility to infection, weakness, poor wound healing and loss of appetite. Smokers and heavy drinkers may benefit from vitamin C supplements.

Fruit and vegetables, especially citrus fruits, blackcurrants, strawberries and kiwi fruit. Raw cabbage, broccoli, peas and potatoes also provide a valuable source.

Extreme deficiency can lead to bone and joint disorders. However, most adults do not need dietary vitamin D supplements, except some elderly people, pregnant women or young children.

Few foods actually contain vitamin D. Those that do include cod liver oil, kippers, mackerel, canned salmon, eggs and milk. Some margerines are fortified with vitamins A and D.

Deficiency is very rare although people with a high intake of polyunsaturates may need more vitamin E to sustain normal cell growth.

Wheatgerm, nuts (particularly peanuts), vegetable oils, eggs, leafy green vegetables and wholemeal bread.

Deficiency may cause brittle bones that break easily (osteoporosis), rickets, muscle problems and heart arrhythmias. Breastfeeding women have an increased need for calcium.

Dairy products such as milk, cheese and yogurt, as well as canned fish, leafy green vegetables, nuts and beans. Reduced fat dairy products contain the same amount of calcium as full-fat varieties.

Deficiency can cause anaemia (a lack of red cell production), which results in dizziness, fatigue and lack of stamina. Some pregnant women may be advised to take supplements.

Meat, chicken, fish (especially pilchards and sardines), liver, kidney, eggs, dried apricots, spinach and other leafy green vegetables, and fortified breakfast cereals.

Deficiency may lead to vomiting, diarrhoea, muscle weakness and loss of appetite. However, excessively high intakes can sometimes cause dangerous toxic effects.

Fruit and vegetables, in particular bananas, apples, carrots, broccoli, dates and oranges. Wholegrain cereals, wheatbran, fish, meat and poultry are also good sources.

Deficiency may arise from dehydration but is rare in Western countries. Excessive sodium can lead to a sustained rise in blood pressure and can also increase the risk of heart disease.

Foods in their natural state do not generally have a high sodium content. However, it is added to many manufactured foods such as bacon, smoked fish, cereals, yeast extract and bread.

Deficiency can sometimes lead to a lack of physical and sexual development, poor wound healing and a loss of appetite.

Seafoods, red meat and offal, dairy products, eggs, some green vegetables and cereals.

FOOD TERMS

ALCOHOL content of different types and volumes of drinks can be measured in units. A unit is equivalent to about 8g or 10ml of pure alcohol. There is approximately 1 unit of alcohol in each of the following:
- ½ pint ordinary strength beer, lager or cider;
- a single 25ml measure of spirits;
- a small glass of wine or sherry;
- a measure of vermouth or aperitif.

Middle-aged and older people who drink small amounts of alcohol on a regular basis appear to be at lower risk of heart disease than non-drinkers. Alcohol may have a protective effect on the heart in two ways – it directly affects the amount of cholesterol carried by the blood and it reduces the likelihood of blood clotting. However, these beneficial effects only apply to men over 40 and women who have been through the menopause, and can be gained by drinking between 1 and 2 units a day. There is no evidence of these beneficial effects in younger people, nor any special benefit from specific drinks (for example, red wine). The health risks for drinkers begin to exceed those of non-drinkers when men drink more than 4 units a day and women drink more than 3 units a day. Government guidelines recommend that men drink no more than 3–4 units a day and women no more than 2–3 units a day for good health. Remember also that alcohol is second only to fat in its calorie content (7kcals/g) and regular drinking may jeopardise weight loss efforts or even cause weight gain.

ANTIOXIDANT VITAMINS such as vitamins C, E and beta-carotene (a form of vitamin A found in fruit and vegetables) are powerful, protective substances that appear to patrol the body, mopping up potentially harmful molecules called free radicals. These free radicals are produced during normal bodily processes, but their production can be increased by environmental pollution, such as cigarette smoke and exhaust fumes. If too many free radicals are left to roam around the body, they may contribute to the development of diseases such as cancer and heart disease. The best way of getting the right mixture and balance of antioxidants is to eat plenty of fruit and vegetables. However, there is no evidence that vitamin and mineral supplements have the same beneficial effect as foods naturally rich in antioxidants. In fact, there is strong evidence that beta-carotene supplements have no protective effect at best and actually increase rates of lung cancer at worst. Beta-carotene supplements should therefore be avoided as a means of protecting against cancer. Other high dose, purified supplements (that contain considerably higher nutrient levels than average intakes from the diet or from one-a-day multi-vitamins) should also be used with caution because they cannot be assumed to be without risk. Always seek medical advice before taking vitamin and mineral supplements.

BLOOD PRESSURE is the pressure exerted by blood on the artery walls. High blood pressure (hypertension) is a risk factor for heart disease. When the heart contracts (systolic pressure) the 'normal' pressure in young healthy adults is about 120mm mercury (Hg). When the heart relaxes (diastolic pressure), the 'normal' pressure is 80mm Hg (written as 120/80). Diastolic blood pressure between 90 and 105 is classified as mild hypertension, between 105 and 120 moderate hypertension, and above 120 is severe hypertension. Blood pressure rises gradually with age so that the average blood pressure of a 65 year old is 160/90. Reducing salt intake, taking regular physical activity, limiting alcohol intake and maintaining a healthy weight can help lower blood pressure levels.

CALORIES are a measure of energy (for example, the energy in food and the amount of energy our bodies need). Kcals is an abbreviation for kilocalories and these are what most people know as calories. KJ is an abbreviation for kilojoules, which are the metric units used to measure energy. Most nutrition labels show figures for kcals and kJs.

There are approximately 4.2kcals in 1kJ, which is why kJ values are always higher.

CARBOHYDRATES are a major source of energy in the diet and should make up at least 50% of the calories we eat. There are two main types of carbohydrate; starches and sugars. Most people need to eat at least half as much again of fibre-rich starchy foods (such as bread, rice, pasta and potatoes) to meet this recommended intake. Sugars can be divided into three different types.

Non-milk extrinsic sugars (NME's) are those not contained within the cellular structure of food or 'added' such as table sugar, confectionery, soft drinks, honey, fruit juices, cakes and biscuits. These sugars are most likely to cause dental caries (see below).

Milk sugars (lactose) are those found in milk and milk products.

Intrinsic sugars are those that are an integral part of the cell structure, such as the sugar in fruit and vegetables. Government healthy eating recommendation states that no more than 11% of the calories we eat should come from NME's, as compared to the current average intake of about 14% of calories. Milk sugars and intrinsic sugars are not as likely to cause dental caries as NME's.

CHOLESTEROL is a type of fat found in animals. It is not essential to eat foods containing cholesterol because it is synthesised by the liver and carried around in the blood by lipoproteins. A high blood cholesterol level can cause atherosclerosis (hardening of the arteries) and is a risk factor for heart disease. Dietary cholesterol (the cholesterol found in foods of animal origin), has very little effect on blood cholesterol levels. However, high intakes of saturated fat increase blood cholesterol levels. Reducing saturated fat intake as part of a healthy diet can help lower raised blood cholesterol levels.

DENTAL CARIES (tooth decay) is the progressive destruction of teeth by acid generated in the bacteria on the tooth surface. The bacteria produce acid as a by-product of the metabolism of dietary sugars and the plaque holds the acid in contact with the tooth like a piece of blotting paper. If sugary foods and drinks (high in NME's, see *Carbohydrates*)

are consumed too often, the acid levels remain high and tooth decay is likely.

DIETARY REFERENCE VALUES have replaced the old Recommended Daily Amounts (RDA's) for nutrients and give you an idea of your requirement of particular nutrients. A range of intakes have now been set for individual nutrients, rather than just one figure. This is because not everybody has the same requirement for nutrients. The new Reference Nutrient Intake (RNI) is the amount of a nutrient that is sufficient for almost all individuals. This level of intake is higher than most people need. The RNI for a range of vitamins and minerals is given below.

NUTRIENT	DAILY RNI	
	Adult men	Adult women
Vitamin A	700mcg	600mcg
Thiamin (B1)	1.0mg	0.8mg
Riboflavin (B2)	1.3mg	1.1mg
Niacin	17mg	13mg
Vitamin B6	1.4mg	1.2mg
Vitamin B12	1.5mcg	1.5mcg
Folate	200mcg	200mcg
Vitamin C	40mg	40mg
Vitamin D	None	None
Vitamin E	>4mg*	>3mg*
Calcium	700mg	700mg
Iron	8.7mg	14.8mg
Potassium	3500mg	3500mg
Selenium	75mcg	60mcg
Zinc	9.5mg	7.0mg

*There is no RNI for vitamin E, but the value given here represents a 'safe daily intake'.

ESSENTIAL FATTY ACIDS
Fat molecules contain units that are called fatty acids. Most fatty acids can be manufactured by the body. However, some polyunsaturated fatty acids cannot be made by the body and have to be supplied by the diet. These are known as essential fatty acids and refer in particular to linoleic acid, alpha linolenic acid and their derivatives. Although the majority of fatty foods contain some essential fatty acids, the richest sources are vegetable and fish oils.

FIBRE (See *Non-starch polysaccharides*)

FLAVONOIDS are compounds that give colour to flowers, fruit and vegetables. Some flavonoids are thought to act as antioxidants and help protect the body from free radical damage (see also *Antioxidant vitamins*).

FREE RADICALS are highly reactive molecules formed during the normal metabolic processes of the body. They cause damage to cells and are thought to provide a biochemical basis for some diseases such as cancer and heart disease. Antioxidants are thought to 'mop-up' free radicals, preventing them from doing harm.

HEART DISEASE and strokes are jointly referred to as 'cardiovascular disease'. Heart disease appears in the form of angina (pains in the arms and/or chest), heart attacks or sudden death. Strokes are usually caused by clots in blood vessels that supply the blood to the brain. The probability of someone suffering from cardiovascular disease is determined by a number of risk factors including age, sex, family history, blood pressure, blood cholesterol and other blood factors, obesity, diabetes, smoking, ethnic group, stress, socio-economic group and physical activity level. Many of these risk factors can be controlled by eating a healthy diet based on the food wheel (see page 6).

MONOUNSATURATES is the name given to a group of fats whose structure consists of carbon atoms linked with only one double bond. Foods containing a high proportion of mononsaturates include olive, rapeseed, fish oils, nuts, milk and some meat and meat products. Replacing saturates in the diet with monounsaturates is thought to lower blood cholesterol levels and reduce the risk of heart disease.

OMEGA-3 FATTY ACIDS is the name given to some of the polyunsaturated fatty acids found particularly in fish oils (for example, cod liver oil). There is evidence to suggest that consuming these fatty acids by eating oily fish (herring, mackerel, trout, salmon, sardines and pilchards) at least once a week can help reduce the risk of blood clots and thereby reduce the risk of heart attacks. These fish oils may help reduce inflammation, which could be of benefit to arthritis patients.

OSTEOPOROSIS is sometimes called 'brittle bone disease' and results in fragile, weak bones that fracture very easily. As children and young adults, bones not only grow but also become more dense as the amount of calcium and other minerals they contain increase. This makes them strong and growth continues until our late 20's or early 30's when bone density reaches its peak. From then on, bones become thinner as we get older. Although this is a normal part of ageing, if peak bone density isn't very high, some people lose more bone than others and this can lead to osteoporosis.

POLYUNSATURATES is the name given to a group of fats whose carbon atoms are joined together by two or more double bonds. They can be divided into two groups known as n-6 and n-3 polyunsaturates according to their structure. The n-6 polyunsaturates are the main type of fat in vegetable oils (sunflower, corn and soyabean), and some meat and meat products. When saturates in the diet are replaced by these polyunsaturates, blood cholesterol levels are reduced. The n-3 polyunsaturates are sometimes called omega-3 fatty acids and are described separately in this Food Terms section.

PHYTOESTROGENS are compounds found in plants that have a mild oestrogen (female sex hormone) activity. Soya products are the major source of phytoestrogens in the diet. Some studies have suggested that diets high in phytoestrogens are associated with low rates of breast cancer. However, as yet there is insufficient evidence to prove this.

PROTEIN is needed in the diet to provide structural material for the growth and repair of tissues. Proteins are also an energy source, and if more protein is consumed than the body needs, the energy is stored as fat. Proteins are large molecules made up of small units called amino acids. When proteins are eaten, they are broken down in the intestines into their constituent amino acids, which are then absorbed. The body then synthesises its own new proteins. Proteins are also used to make hormones and other chemical messengers. There are 20 different amino acids found in plant and animal proteins, but the body has a limited capacity to convert one amino acid into another. Some amino acids cannot be made from others and have to be supplied by the diet. These are called essential amino acids. Protein 'quality' refers to the fact that certain foods (for example, those of animal origin including meat, milk and eggs) contain amino acids in similar proportions to those found in the human body and are therefore used efficiently by the body. Foods of plant origin, (for example cereals and beans) have a low protein 'quality' when eaten separately. But when eaten together (such as beans on toast) the protein 'quality' is as good as foods of animal origin. For most people, protein quality is not worth worrying about, because protein is abundant in most of the foods we eat. Children given a vegetarian diet need a good mix of plant proteins to give them the high quality protein they need for growth and development. The RNI (see *Dietary Reference Values*) for protein intake in adults is 45g per day for women and 55g per day for man.

SATURATES is the name given to a group of fats whose carbon atoms are linked together by single bonds. A high proportion of saturates can be found in foods such as milk and dairy products, meat and meat products, spreads, cooking fats, biscuits, cakes and pastries. High intakes of saturates are directly related to increased levels of blood cholesterol (and therefore heart disease risk). Intake of saturates has fallen from 19% of food energy in 1989 to 16% of food energy in 1992. According to current healthy eating guidelines, saturates should provide no more than 10% of the calories we eat.

TRANS FATTY ACIDS have a slightly different structure to other unsaturated fatty acids and high intakes are thought to have the similar undesirable effects on blood cholesterol levels as saturates. This caused concern some years ago when it was discovered that many of the fat spreads people were eating as a replacement for butter where high in trans fats. This is because trans fats were produced during the industrial process of hardening oil used in the manufacture of margarines and spreads. However, most polyunsaturated and monounsaturated margarines now contain minimal amounts. Trans fats are naturally present in some foods such as butter, milk and meat. It is recommended that no more than 2% of the calories we eat should come from trans fats.

NON-STARCH POLYSACCHARIDES is the technical name for dietary fibre. It includes soluble and insoluble fibre. Soluble fibre can be found in oats, pulses and fruits and vegetables. It may help reduce high blood cholesterol levels if consumed as part of a healthy diet that is low in saturates. Insoluble fibre is the type found in cereals (bread, pasta, breakfast cereals, rice), especially wholewheat/wholegrain varieties. It can prevent and reduce the symptoms of constipation and may also reduce the risk of other bowel disorders, diverticular disease and possibly colon cancer. High fibre foods tend to be low in fat and have the added bonus of filling you up using relatively few calories. Healthy eating guidelines recommend we eat 18g fibre a day. This is 6g more than the current average intake.

SODIUM CHLORIDE is the chemical name for salt. The RNI (see *Dietary reference values*) for salt is 1.6g/day, which meets the majority of people's needs for sodium. This is equivalent to about 1g of salt per day. However, the current average intake of salt is about 9g per day. This level of intake may lead to raised blood pressure in some people – a risk factor for heart disease. Current dietary guidelines recommend that salt intake be cut by at least a third to 6g per day. This is still in excess of physiological requirements, but is a practical intake to aim for in the short term. In the UK, 65–85% of the salt eaten comes from manufactured foods, over which consumers have little control. However, reducing the salt added during cooking and at the table will help to reduce intakes as would choosing fewer processed and ready-made foods.

NUTRITION LABELLING

Reading nutrition labels can tell you a lot about the food you are eating, which is important if you want to eat a healthy, balanced diet. But understanding the information can be tricky, so here's a brief guide to help you.

Food packets contain a great deal of information about the food inside but they can sometimes be confusing or even misleading. You can often learn something about the food from its name. Certain foods are required by law to be sold under prescribed names, such as margarine, ice cream and bread, which contain specified quantities of ingredients. The manufacturer is also required to state a contact name and address, and list the food's country of origin, which can either mean the country in which the food was grown or in which it was packaged.

What a nutrition label tells you

Regulations require that any packaged foods displaying a nutritional claim (for example, 'low fat'), must also display nutrition labelling. If no claim is made on the packaging then manufacturers do not have to show nutrition information. Nutrition labels have to show the amount of energy, protein, carbohydrate and fat in 100g of the food. Values for sugar, saturated fat, fibre and sodium are also sometimes given. Labels making specific claims have to show values for the nutrient about which the claim is made.

Nutrition Information

Typical Values	Per ½pizza	Per 100g (3.5oz)
Energy	2316kJ	1158kJ
	550kcals	275kcals
Protein	25.0g	12.5g
Carbohydrate	70.8g	35.4g
of which sugars	5.2g	2.6g
of which starch	65.6g	32.8g

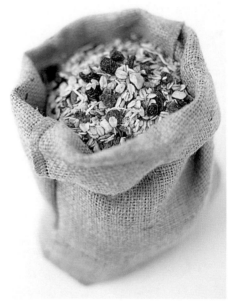

Fat	18.6g	9.3g
of which saturates	6.8g	3.4g
Monounsaturates	6.4g	3.2g
Polyunsaturates	4.6g	2.3g
Fibre	3.4g	1.7g
Sodium	1.4g	0.7g

* For definitions of the above nutrients see Food Terms on pages 12–15.

Ingredients list

Ingredients are listed by weight – the one present in the largest amount appears first and others are listed in descending order (except water). You can use ingredients lists to compare products for value or to help you avoid ingredients you don't want to eat.

Per serving or per 100g

Although it's often more useful to have nutrition values 'per serving' of food, manufacturers have to give values per 100g as well. This is useful for comparing the nutrient content of two different foods. You can still calculate the nutrient content of a portion by multiplying the amounts in 100g by the weight of your portion (g)/100.

The weight of the food in a package is usually given on the label accompanied by a big e (for example, 250ml e). This means that the average quantity of food must be accurate, but that the weight of each packet may vary slightly.

Nutrition claims

There are voluntary guidelines that most food manufacturers and retailers use to govern the exact meaning of some nutrition claims. However, not all claims are covered by these guidelines and not all food manufacturers stick to them when they are. Claims can also be quite misleading. For example if a product says 'reduced fat' this means that it should contain at least 25% less fat than the standard product, but in the case of biscuits or crisps, for example the product is likely still to be relatively high in fat. The only way to be sure is to read the nutrition label. Here's what some of the common claims should mean:

Claim	Meaning
'low fat' or 'low sugar'	No more than 5g of fat or sugar per 100g food.
'low saturates'	No more than 3g saturated fat per 100g food.
'reduced fat' or 'reduced sugar'	The product must contain at least 25% less fat or sugar than the standard product.
'low sodium'	No more than 40mg per 100g.
'high fibre'	More than 6g per 100g.
'fat free'	No more than 0.15g per 100g.

'saturates free'	No more than 0.1g per 100g.
'sugar free'	No more than 0.2g per 100g.
'no added sugar'	No sugars or foods composed mainly of sugars (for example, dried fruit or concentrated fruit juice) should be added to the food or any of its ingredients.

The following claims are not covered by voluntary government guidelines and may mean something different each time, the only way to be really sure is by checking the label:

Light or Lite: this could mean light in weight, light in colour or more often low in fat.

Half fat: this means that the food contains half the fat of its standard counterpart.

Lower fat: this usually means that the food contains less fat than its standard counterpart, but how much lower can only be ascertained by reading the labels. The chances are, it's not that much lower otherwise it would be covered by the 'low fat' or 'reduced fat' claim.

Virtually fat free: this usually means there is very little fat in a food. But remember, if a label says '90% fat free' it also means it contains 10% fat, which means that the product can't be classified as low fat!

'Diet' products

According to food labelling regulations the word 'diet' can only appear on products that make a 'low calorie' claim. To classify as a low calorie food, a food must contain no more than 40 calories per 100g or 100ml (in the case of drinks) or per serving if less than 100g. The claim must also be accompanied by the statement '...can help slimming or weight control only as part of a calorie controlled diet.'

FOOD	CARB	FIBRE	FAT	ENERGY	
	g	g	g	kcal	kJ

ALCOHOL
Beers
ale, brown, bottled – small, 275ml	8.3	0	0	82	346
ale, pale, bottled – small, 275ml	5.5	0	0	77	325
ale, strong – small, 275ml	17	0	0	182	756
beer, average, 1 pint, 574ml	13	0	0	182	756
beer, bitter, canned, 440ml	10.3	0	0	143	586
beer, bitter, canned, large, 500ml	11.6	0	0	161	660
beer, bitter, low alcohol, 1 pint, 574ml	12	0	0	75	310
beer, draught, 1 pint, 574ml	13.3	0	0	184	755
beer, keg, 1 pint, 574ml	13.2	0	0	178	741
beer, mild, draught, 1 pint, 574ml	9.3	0	0	145	597
lager, average, canned and draught, 500ml	Tr	0	0	145	605
lager, bottled, large, 500ml	7.5	0	0	146	598
lager, reduced-alcohol, 1 pint, 574ml	8.6	0	0	57.4	235
lager, premium, strong, 500ml	Tr	0	0	295	1220
shandy, canned, large, 500ml	15	0	0	55	240
stout, bottled, small, 275ml	11.4	0	0	100	429
stout, strong, large, 500ml	10.5	0	0	195	817
stout, strong, small, 275ml	5.8	0	0	107	449

Ciders
cider, dry, 1 pint, 574ml	15	0	0	208	873
cider, sweet, 1 pint, 574ml	24.4	0	0	244	1011
cider, vintage, strong, 1 pint, 574ml	42	0	0	578	2417

Cocktails
cocktail, Bloody Mary, 165ml	5.5	0.5	0	124	520
cocktail, Daiquiri, 60ml	4	0	0	111	465
cocktail, Tequila Sunrise, 60ml	7	0	0	66	275

Liqueurs
liqueur, egg-based, 25ml	7	0	1.6	65	273
liqueur, cherry brandy/coffee, 25ml	8.2	0	0	65.5	275
liqueur, cream, 25ml	6	0	4	81	338
liqueur, drambuie, 25ml	6.1	0	0	78.5	330

Spirits
spirits, average, 40% volume – brandy, gin, rum, vodka, whiskey, 25ml	0	0	0	55	230
spirits, average, 37.5% volume, 25ml	0	0	0	51	214

Wines
wine, red, small glass, 120ml	0.4	0	0	85	356
wine, rose, 120ml	3.1	0	0	89	367
wine, white, dry, 120ml	0.7	0	0	82	343
wine, white, medium, 120ml	4.3	0	0	94	388
wine, white, sweet, 120ml	7.4	0	0	118	493
wine, fortified, port, 50ml	6	0	0	80	327
wine, fortified, sherry, dry, 50ml	0.7	0	0	58	240
wine, fortified, sherry, medium, 50ml	3	0	0	60	252
wine, fortified, sherry, sweet, 50ml	3.5	0	0	68	284
wine, fortified, vermouth, dry, 50ml	1.5	0	0	55	227

ALCOHOL Drinking alcohol in moderate amounts (no more than 2 to 3 units a day for women, or 3 to 4 units for men), does not appear to have any adverse health effects in adults of a healthy weight. However, do have at least one or two alcohol-free days a week and avoid binge drinking. Try to limit alcohol to meal times.

BEER A drink made by the fermentation of cereals (usually barley), beer can be high in calories and may also weaken resolve when it comes to reaching for high-fat snacks.

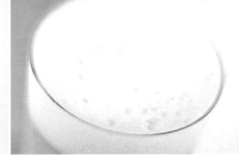

RECIPE For a refreshing summer drink with just 65 calories, pour about 60ml of dry sparkling wine and 60ml of soda water over berries and allow to stand for a few minutes.

WHITE WINE Mix with ice-cold soda water to make a wine spritzer with half the calories of a glass of wine.

SPIRITS Adding full-sugar mixers or juice to a spirit increases the calorie content. Try diet mixers or soda water for a change.

FOOD	CARB	FIBRE	FAT	ENERGY	
	g	g	g	kcal	kJ
ALCOHOL CONT.					
wine, fortified, vermouth, sweet, 50ml	7.6	0	0	75	315
champagne, 125ml	1.7	0	0	95	394
APPLE					
chutney, 1 serving, 35g	18	0.6	0	68	288
cooking, stewed with sugar, 4oz, 100g	19	1.8	0	74	314
cooking, stewed without sugar, 4oz, 100g	8	2	0	33	138
eating, raw, unpeeled, 1 average, 5oz, 125g	13	2.2	0	52.5	224
eating, raw, peeled, 1 average, 4oz, 100g	11	0	0	45	190
dried, 1oz, 25g	15	2.4	0	60	254
juice, unsweeted, small glass, 4fl oz, 100ml	10	Tr	0	38	164
juice, concentrated, 1fl oz, 25g	14	Tr	0	57	243
APRICOT					
canned in juice, 6 halves, 120g	9.6	1.2	0	41	176
canned in syrup, 6 halves, 120g	19	1.2	0	76	321
raw, 3, 110g	6.8	2	0	28	119
stewed with sugar, 4oz serving, 100g	18	2	0	72	308
stewed without sugar, 4oz serving, 100g	6	2	0	27	115
dried, 3 whole, 50g	22	4	0	94	401
ready to eat – semi-dried, 4oz, 100g	36	6.3	0	158	674
juice drink, 35% juice, 1 glass, 250ml	20	1	0	18	75
nectar, 50% juice, glass, 250ml	32	0	0	129	540
ARTICHOKE					
globe, boiled, 1 medium, 220g	2.6	1	0	17	70
hearts, canned in brine, drained, 1 heart, 50g	1	1.5	0	8	35
Jerusalem, peeled, boiled, 1 medium, 100g	10	3.5	0	41	207
ASPARAGUS					
canned, drained, 8 spears, 100g	1.5	2.9	0	24	100
fresh, boiled, 4 spears, 120g	1	1	0	15	63
AUBERGINE (see also EGGPLANT)					
fried in corn oil, 100g	2.8	2.3	32	302	1262
raw, 100g	2.2	2	0.4	15	64
AVOCADO					
medium, 1 raw 100g	1.9	3.4	19.5	190	784
BABY FOOD					
baby rusk, plain, average, 100g	82.8	N	7.9	408	1729
rusk, flavoured, 100g	78.1	N	9	401	1698
rusk, low sugar, 100g	77.8	N	9.7	414	1751
rusk, wholemeal, 100g	76.5	N	10.1	411	1739
cereal, ground muesli, 100g	70	N	8	400	1690
cereal, creamed porridge,100g	58	N	5.5	360	1510
cereal, mixed, powder, 100g	71	N	5	377	1599
cereal, fruit, banana & apple, powder, 100g	70	N	3.8	359	1527
cereal, apple & blackberry, powder, 100g	77	N	4	365	1552
baby rice, powder, 100g	78	N	3	365	1553
baby rice, mixed, 100g	78	N	2	372	1565
dessert, creamed rice, jar, 128g	8	0	0.5	40	155
dessert, fruit, powder, 100g	90	1.3	0.6	383	1635

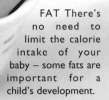

FAT There's no need to limit the calorie intake of your baby – some fats are important for a child's development.

BEST FOR BABY Breast or formula milk is the only food that babies need for the first 4–6 months. Breast milk is particularly ideal because it provides all the necessary nutrients, together with certain antibodies that help protect young babies from infection.

BABY FOOD Most babies are

ready for 'solid' foods by about the age of 4 months. Keep things simple to start with, by offering pureed fruit or vegetables, with no added salt or sugar. Try to keep commercially produced baby foods to a minimum, and always check labels to ensure that the food is suitable for your child.

FIBRE Babies only have small stomachs and need to obtain a lot of nutrients from small portions. Foods high in fibre such as wholewheat cereals and/or wholemeal bread can be filling, without providing sufficient energy, so avoid offering them every day.

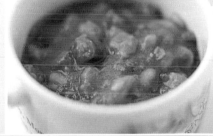

RECIPE To make a nutritious and tasty 'first food' for your baby, steam some swede (or pumpkin) and potato until tender. Purée and add a little breast or formula milk and then pass through a sieve in order to remove any lumps.

FOOD	CARB	FIBRE	FAT	ENERGY	
	g	g	g	kcal	kJ
BABY FOOD CONT.					
dessert, caramel custard, 100g	13	N	2.5	82	345
dessert, fruit custard, 100g	17	N	0.5	74	310
dinner, beef, junior, 100g	10	I	0.5	60	240
dinner, chicken & vegetable, 100g	8	1.5	1.5	60	250
dinner, chicken, junior, 100g	9	0.5	I	55	230
dinner, chicken noodle, junior, 100g	9.5	0.5	I	57	240
egg/cheese based meal, canned, 100g	10	I	3.4	82	344
meat based meal, average, canned, 100g	8.6	1.1	3	73	306
dinner, lamb casserole, jar 200g	18	N	2	121	510
dinner, lamb, junior, 100g	7	I	2.5	62	260
dinner, lentil hot-pot, jar, 200g	20	N	0.5	114	480
dinner, fish based, average, canned, 100g	9	0.6	3	76	321
dinner, garden vegetable, jar, 200g	24	N	0.5	124	520
dinner, mixed vegetable, strained, 100g	8.5	N	I	46	195
dinner, pasta & vegetable, jar, 200g	27	N	I	138	580
dinner, pasta based, average, canned, 100g	8.5	0.7	3	71	300
dinner, vegetable based, canned, 100g	10	2	2	67	284
BACON					
bits, 2tsp	0	0	1.5	30	125
fried & 2 fried eggs	0	0	18	215	905
middle rasher, fried, 1 slice, 10g	0	0	3	37	155
middle rasher, trimmed, fried, 1, 10g	0	0	I	23	95
middle rasher, grilled, 1, 10g	0	0	2	32	135
middle rasher, trimmed, grilled, 1, 10g	0	0	I	24	100
BAGEL					
plain, average, 1, 60g	29	+	0.5	137	575
BAKLAVA					
bought, average piece, 100g	40	+	17.5	322	1349
BAMBOO SHOOTS					
canned or bottled, drained, 1 cup, 140g	1.5	2.2	0	11	45
raw, 50g	3	N	0	14.3	60
BANANA					
chips, crystallised, 1oz, approx. 25 chips, 25g	15	0.5	7.8	128	534
dried, 100g	28	3	0	119	500
raw, peeled, 140g	32.5	I	Tr	133	564
BARLEY					
bran, raw, 40g	30	+	I	131	550
cooked, 1 portion, 180g	38	+	1.5	190	800
pearl, cooked, 100g	27.7	+	I	120	510
wholegrain, raw, 100g	64	15	2	301	1282
BEANS & LENTILS					
aduki, cooked, 4oz portion, 100g	22.5	5.5	0.2	123	525
baked, canned in tomato sauce, 100g	15	3.5	0.6	81	345
balor, canned in salted water, 100g	2.8	2.7	0.1	19	83
black-eyed, cooked, 100g	20	3.5	0.7	116	494
black gram, cooked, 100g	13.5	N	0.4	89	379
black kidney, cooked, 100g	24.5	N	0.5	130	545

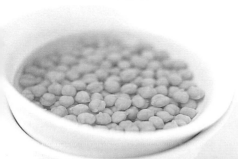

KIDNEY BEANS Next time you make chilli con carne, try using more kidney beans and less beef mince, as kidney beans are high in fibre and supply all the protein of meat without the fat.

CHICKPEAS Readily available in tins, chickpeas are a great source of fibre and a cheap, low-fat alternative to meat.

BEANS Rich in protein, dietary fibre and complex carbohydrates, and low in fat, beans should be an essential part of our diet, especially for people who don't eat any or much meat. The canned varieties are great if you don't have time to soak dried beans overnight.

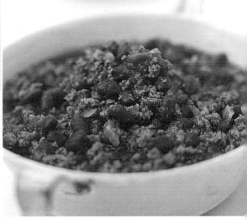

SOYA BEANS An excellent source of phytoestrogens (compounds which may have some beneficial effects in menopausal women), soya beans also provide the best quality protein of all the pulses.

RECIPE Process chickpeas with a little tahini, garlic, lemon juice, oil and water to make a delicious low-fat dip. Serve with pieces of wholemeal bread or warmed pitta bread.

FOOD	CARB.	FIBRE	FAT	ENERGY	
	g	g	g	kcal	kJ
BEANS AND LENTILS CONT.					
borlotti, canned, drained, 100g	25	N	0.5	112	470
borlotti, cooked, 100g	28.5	N	0.5	146	612
broad, fresh, cooked, 100g	5.6	5.4	0.8	48	204
butter (cannellini), canned, 100g	13	4.6	0.5	77	327
chickpeas, canned, drained, 100g portion	16	4.1	2.9	115	487
green, fresh, cooked, 100g	3	2.4	0	22	92
green, frozen, cooked, 100g	4.7	4.1	0	25	108
haricot, cooked, 100g	17.2	6.1	0.5	95	406
kidney, red, canned, drained, cooked, 100g	12.2	4.1	0.5	70	380
lentils, canned in tomato sauce, 100g	9.3	1.7	0.2	55	236
lentils, red, split, cooked, 100g	17.5	2	0.4	100	424
lentils, whole, dried, cooked, 100g	17	3.8	0.7	105	446
lima, dried, cooked, 100g	10	5.5	Tr	70	295
mung, cooked, 100g	15.3	10	0.4	91	389
pinto, cooked, 100g	24	N	0.7	137	583
red kidney bean, cooked, 100g	17.4	6.7	0.5	103	440
red kidney beans, in chilli sauce, 100g	13.1	3.6	2.6	91	383
runner, fresh, cooked, 100g	2.3	1.9	0.5	18	76
soya, canned, drained, 100g	5.1	6.1	7.3	141	590
soya, canned in tomato sauce, 100g	7	3	3	90	380
soya, dried, cooked, 100g	1.5	6.1	7.5	128	540
three-bean mix, canned, drained, 100g	14	N	0.5	86	360
tofu, soya bean, steamed, 100g	0.7	N	4.2	73	304
BEEF					
steak, lean, grilled, 1 medium, 117g	0	0	10.5	224	940
steak, untrimmed, grilled, 1, 120g	0	0	12.5	250	1040
chuck steak, untrimmed, simmered, 1, 190g	0	0	26	486	2040
corned, canned, 100g	0	0	12.5	217	905
corned, sliced, 100g	0	0	9	150	625
fillet steak, lean, grilled, 1, small, 85g	0	0	7	167	700
fillet steak, untrimmed, grilled, 1 small, 85g	0	0	11	198	830
Beef burgers, grilled, 100g	0.1	0	24.4	326	1355
homemade, 100g	1	0	20	287	1194
takeaway, in bun with salad, 100g	18	N	12.7	238	996
economy, frozen, grilled, 100g	9.7	0.8	19.3	273	1138
heart, simmered, 100g	0	0	5.9	179	752
kidney, simmered, 100g	0	0	6.1	153	641
liver, simmered, 100g	0	0	9.5	198	831
mince, simmered, drained, 170g	0	0	20.5	390	1623
mince, lean, simmered, drained, 170g	0	0	16.5	309	1300
oxtail, simmered, 100g	0	0	13.5	243	1014
pepper steak with cream sauce, 1 serving, 200g	0	0	35	536	2250
pie, bought, family size, 1 serving, 250g	38.5	+	36.5	560	2355
pie, bought, individual, 250g	45	+	34.5	564	2370
pie, bought, party size, 1, 40g	7.5	+	7.5	111	465
rib steak, lean, grilled, 100g	0	0	5.5	176	740
rissoles, fried, 2, 340g	0	+	30	662	2780

CASSEROLES To make your casseroles lower in calories but still full of flavour, prepare one day in advance and refrigerate overnight. Before reheating, carefully lift off and discard the fat that will have risen and set on the surface.

MINCE To make really lean mince, buy lean steak and mince it yourself in a food processor. Alternatively, buy extra lean mince, cook without fat and drain off all juices.

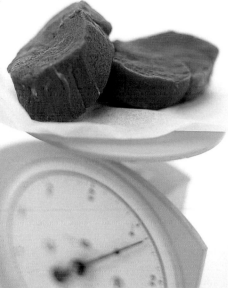

BEEF Lean beef, cooked without any added fat, can contain as little as 5% fat. Moderate amounts of red meat, such as beef, can be part of a healthy balanced diet and is an excellent source of iron and other minerals. Choose lean cuts that have had all visible fat removed and use low-fat marinades, such as lemon juice, mustard, soy sauce and herbs.

RECIPE To give a fillet steak extra flavour when you are grilling or frying it without fat, baste with a little marinade of soy sauce, spread both sides with wholegrain mustard or coat in cracked black pepper.

COOKING To avoid adding extra fat, cook your meat on a lightly oiled griddle pan or barbecue, but don't turn the meat too often and allow to rest before serving to keep it from drying out.

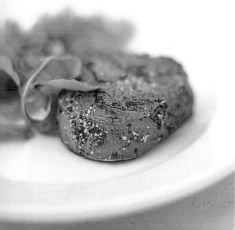

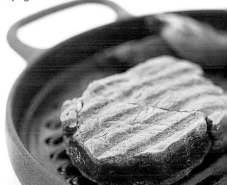

FOOD	CARB	FIBRE	FAT	ENERGY	
	g	g	g	kcal	kJ
BEEF CONT.					
round steak, lean, grilled, 100g	0	0	6	176	740
round steak, untrimmed, grilled, 100g	0	0	9.5	202	850
rump steak, lean, grilled, 175g	0	0	11.5	334	1405
rump steak, untrimmed, grilled, 200g	0	0	33.5	538	2260
silverside, lean, baked, 2 slices, 80g	0	0	3.5	131	550
silverside, untrimmed, baked, 2 slices, 85g	0	0	10	189	795
sirloin steak, lean, grilled, 110g	0	0	9.5	192	806
sirloin steak, untrimmed, grilled, 127g	0	0	24	348	1460
skirt steak, lean, simmered, 100g	0	0	5	188	790
skirt steak, untrimmed, simmered, 100g	0	0	6	196	825
steak, lean, grilled, 1 small, 110g	0	0	9	216	910
steak, untrimmed, grilled, 1 small, 130g	0	0	20.5	330	1390
T-bone, lean, grilled, 100g	0	0	5.5	134	565
T-bone, untrimmed, grilled, 100g	0	0	8	164	690
tongue, simmered, 100g	0	0	25	307	1290
topside roast, lean, baked, 2 slices. 80g	0	0	4	124	520
topside roast, untrimmed, baked, 2 slices, 90g	0	0	9	171	720
topside steak, lean, grilled,1 small, 100g	0	0	5	151	635
topside steak, untrimmed, grilled, 1 small,100g	0	0	6.5	162	680
tripe, simmered, 100g	0	0	3	83	350
BEETROOT					
fresh, peeled, boiled, 2 slices	5	0.4	0	25	105
pickled, 5 slices, 100g	14	1.7	0	64	270
raw, grated, 30g	2.5	0.6	0	12	50
BISCUITS					
assorted creams, 1, 15g	12.5	N	4	75	315
brandy snaps, 1, 10g	6.4	Tr	2	44	183
bourbon, 1, 12.5g	8.5	N	3.2	64	270
chocolate, full coated, 1 small, 25g	17	0.6	7	131	549
chocolate coated, 2, 30g	20	0.9	7.2	148	621
chocolate chip cookies, 1	4.5	N	2	36	150
chocolate shortbreads, 1	5	N	2.5	35	147
choc-chip, 1, 10g	8	N	2	51	215
cookies, 1, 10g	9	N	2.5	62	260
coconut ice, 1	9.5	+	3.5	71	300
cream biscuit, 1, 10g	6.4	N	2	46	194
custard cream, 1, 12.5g	8	N	3	64	270
digestive biscuits, plain, 2, 30g	20	0.7	6.3	141	593
digestive biscuit, chocolate, 1, 15g	10	0.3	3.6	74	311
flapjacks, 1, 25g	15	0.7	6.5	121	552
ginger nuts, 2, 20g	16	0.4	3	91	385
gingernut biscuits, homemade, 1, 20g	13	0.3	3.4	90	377
golden oat, 1, 15g	9.5	0.5	1.5	54	225
jaffa cake, 2	7	N	1	36	153
melting moments, 1, 10g	5.5	0.1	3.6	55	229
oatcakes, homemade, 1, 10g	6.3	0.6	1.8	44.5	187
oatcakes, retail, 1, 10g	6.3	N	1.8	44	185

BISCUITS Sweet biscuits are often high in sugar and saturated fat, but they can be useful as a quick source of carbohydrate. If you want something lower in fat to snack on, reach for fresh or dried fruit, or a crispbread or rice cake with cottage cheese. Alternatively, baking your own biscuits will help you cut back on fat and sugar.

SHORTBREAD High in fat and sugar, that lovely melt-in-the-mouth texture comes from the high ratio of butter to flour.

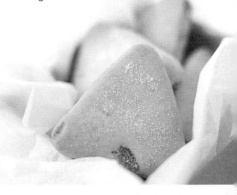

COOKIES Chewy ones get their texture from the high amount of butter and sugar. Don't be fooled into thinking oatmeal biscuits are lower in fat, though they do contain more fibre.

BISCOTTI A great low-fat biscuit. Made with eggs, they contain no butter and they also have extra fibre because they contain nuts.

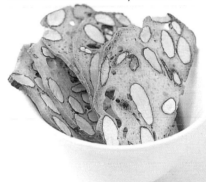

CREAM-FILLED High in fat and sugar, the centre is usually a mix of icing sugar, butter and water, and in most cases the biscuit is sweet and buttery.

LOW-FAT There are biscuits now available in supermarkets that are up to 70% lower in fat than normal biscuits but they are still relatively high in fat and sugar.

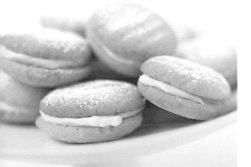

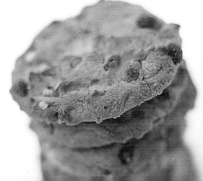

FOOD	CARB	FIBRE	FAT	ENERGY	
	g	g	g	kcal	kJ
BISCUITS CONT.					
fruit slice, 1, 15g	8	+	0.5	37	155
sandwich biscuit, 2, 25g	17.3	N	6.5	128	538
semi-sweet, 2, 15g	11.2	0.3	2.5	69	289
semi-sweet, coconut type, 1, 10g	9	0.1	2	56	23
semi-sweet, morning coffee type, 1, 12g	4.5	0.1	1	30	126
semi-sweet, rich tea type, 1, 7.5g	5.6	0.1	1.2	35	145
short-sweet biscuit, 2, 20g	12.4	0.3	4.7	94	393
shortbread, 2 fingers, 35g	22	0.8	9	174	730
shortbread, cream, 1	10.5	0	4.5	87	365
shortbread, scotch finger, 1	12	0.5	4	88	370
shortcake, 2, 20g	12	0.3	5	94	393
wafers, filled, 3, 18g	12	N	5.4	96	404
savoury, biscuit, 1	2	N	0.5	14	60
savoury, crackers, cream, 3, 21g	14.3	0.6	3.4	92	390
savoury, crackers, wholemeal, 3, 21g	15	1	2.4	87	366
crispbread, cracotte type, 3, 15g	9.4	0.4	2.3	61	256
crispbread, rye, 3, 24g	17	2.8	0.5	77	328
matzos, 1, 30g	26	1	0.6	115	490
oatcakes, 2, 26g	16.4	1.2	4.8	115	482
water biscuits, 3, 21g	16	0.6	2.6	92	390
BLACKBERRIES					
canned, sweetened, 100g	23	+	0	92	385
fresh, raw, ½ punnet, 100g	12.5	3.1	0.5	52	220
frozen, 100g	15.5	+	0.5	64	270
BLACKCURRANT JUICE					
prepared, diluted, 250ml	28	0	0	107	450
BLUEBERRIES					
canned in syrup, drained, 100g	17	+	0	69	290
frozen, 100g	12	+	0.5	51	215
raw, ½ punnet, 100g	14	1.8	0.5	56	235
BOYSENBERRIES					
canned in heavy syrup, 100g	22.5	2.6	0	88	370
canned, no added sugar, 100g	4	+	0	27	115
raw, ½ punnet, 100g	6	+	0	13	55
BRAN (see CEREAL)					
BRANDY BUTTER					
1 tbsp, 30g	16	0	8	146	615
BRAWN					
2 slices, 70g	0	0	12	151	635
BREAD					
bagel, plain, average, 1, 60g	29	+	0.5	137	575
breadcrumbs, homemade, 100g	77.5	2.2	1.9	354	1508
breadcrumbs, manufactured, 100g	78.5	N	2.1	354	1505
brown bread, average, 38g	16.8	1.3	0.8	83	352
brown roll, crusty, 48g	24.2	1.7	1.3	122	521
brown roll, soft, 48g	24.9	1.7	1.8	129	547
chapatis, made with fat, 1, 100g	48.3	N	12.8	328	1383

FLAVOURED CRACKERS These can be high in fat and salt, so always check the nutrition label for full information.

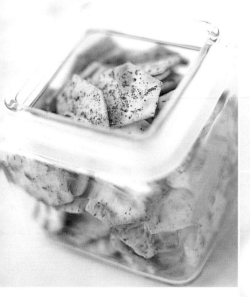

BISCUITS, CRACKERS & CRISPBREADS

Some savoury biscuits, such as rice crackers and oatcakes, are low in fat and sugar, and make a good alternative to bread. However, be aware that some savoury biscuits can be high in fat and salt. Choose wholewheat or high fibre varieties to boost your fibre intake.

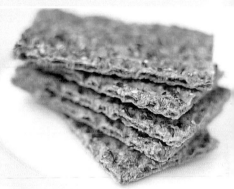

WATER CRACKERS Relatively fat-free, these crackers are a good source of carbohydrate. Serve them with low-fat soft cheese or yogurt dips, salad vegetables or reduced fat hummus.

CRISPBREADS A high-fibre choice for an afternoon snack. Top with some cottage or low-fat soft cheese and slices of ripe tomato.

RICE CRACKERS A tasty low-fat cracker that provides a handy gluten-free snack high in carbohydrate.

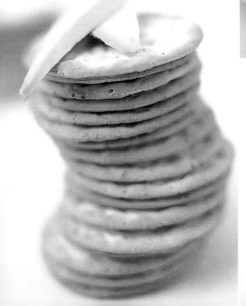

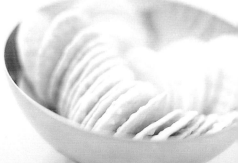

FOOD	CARB	FIBRE	FAT	ENERGY	
	g	g	g	kcal	kJ
BREAD CONT.					
chapatis, made without fat, 1, 100g	43.7	N	1	202	860
corn, 90g	20	+	7	178	750
croissant, 60g	23	1	12.2	216	903
crumpet, wholemeal, toasted, 1, 44g	17	1.5	0.5	84	355
currant bread, 1 slice, 25g	12.7	+	1.9	72	305
focaccia, 1, 50g	30	2	1.5	139	585
focaccia, herb & garlic, 1, 70g	32	2	1.5	170	715
granary, 1 slice, 38g	17.6	1.6	1	89	380
hamburger roll, 85g	41.5	1.3	4.3	224	953
loaf, average, white, 2 slices	35	3.5	2	189	795
loaf, fruit, fruit & spice, 2 slices	34.5	+	2	177	745
loaf, fruit, raisin toast, 2 slices	26	+	1.5	134	565
loaf, fruit, spicy fruit, 2 slices	33.5	+	2	174	730
loaf, gluten/wheat free, 2 slices	12	+	2	64	270
loaf, mixed grain, 2 slices	33.5	+	3.5	196	825
loaf, multi-grains, 2 slices	35	+	2	187	785
loaf, pumpernickel, 2 slices	18	3.7	1	92	385
loaf, rice bran, 2 slices	2	+	10	69	290
loaf, black rye, 1 slice	42	+	2	214	900
loaf, rye, 2 slices	30	2.2	3	176	740
loaf, soya & linseed, 2 slices	40	++	6	259	1090
malt bread, 1 slice, 35g	19.9	+	0.8	94	399
naan, 1, 160g	80	3	20	538	2264
papadum, fried, 1, 13g	5.1	N	2.2	48	201
pitta, white, 1, 95g	55	2.1	1.1	252	1071
rye bread, 25g	11.4	1.1	0.4	55	233
soda bread, yeast-free, 1, 60g	35	1.2	1.5	178	750
toasted, regular, 1, 45g	19.5	1	0.5	93	390
tortillas made with wheat flour, 1, 30g	15	0.8	2	86	360
wheatgerm bread, 1 slice, 25g	10.9	0.8	0.8	57	244
white bread, average, 35g	17.3	0.5	0.7	82	357
white bread med. slice, large loaf, 36g	16.8	0.5	0.5	78	333
white bread roll, crusty, 1, 50g	28.8	0.8	1.1	140	596
white bread roll, soft, 1, 45g	23.2	0.7	1.9	121	512
white bread, fried in oil, 45g	21.8	0.7	14.3	226	946
white bread, with added fibre, 1 slice, 38g	17.4	1.1	0.5	81	342
wholemeal bread, average, 38g	15.8	2.2	0.9	82	347
wholemeal roll, 1 average, 48g	23.2	2.8	1.4	116	492
wholemeal, roll, 1 large, 105g	46	6	2.5	250	1050
stick, French (baguette), white, 1, 50g	22.5	0.7	1.5	128	540
stick, French (baguette), wholemeal, 1, 50g	21	+	1.5	119	500
toast, French, 2 slices	20	+	8.5	182	765
BROCCOLI					
raw, 100g	0	2.6	0	24	100
BRUSSEL SPROUTS					
raw, 100g	2	4.1	0	24	100

WHITE A good source of carbohydrate, fibre, vitamins and minerals. It contains less fibre than wholemeal varities, but is still low in fat and an important part of a healthy diet.

WHOLEMEAL AND MIXED GRAIN Both have more fibre and vitamins than white bread, with wholemeal having the most.

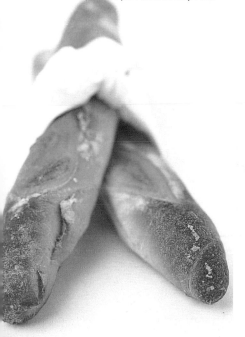

BREAD

Let's dispel the myth once and for all that bread is fattening — it is the spreads that we cover it with that can be. Bread provides us with dietary fibre, energy and valuable vitamins and minerals, and even white bread is nutritious. One pitfall is that commercial bread can be high in sodium — check the label for details.

HI-FIBRE A flour with added fibre, which gives it the same amount of fibre as wholemeal. Perfect for school packed lunches.

RYE Light rye has a similar nutritional value to white bread, whereas dark or black rye is a better source of fibre, iron and magnesium.

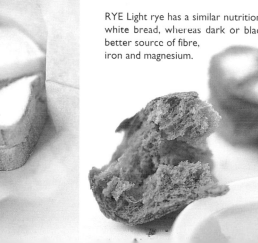

FOOD	CARB	FIBRE	FAT	ENERGY	
	g	g	g	kcal	kJ
BUCKWHEAT KERNELS					
boiled, 100g	73	2.1	2.5	334	1400
BULGUR (Cracked Wheat)					
cooked, 100g	68.5	+	2.5	319	1340
BUN					
brioche, 1	N	N	16	278	1170
cinnamon, 1, 100g	45	1.5	15	263	1105
chelsea, 78g	43.8	1.3	10.8	285	1203
cream, 1 small, 60g	15.5	0.5	21.5	261	1082
finger, iced, 1, 65g	30	N	5	192	805
fruit, iced, 1, 90g	42	N	7	265	1115
hot cross, 1, 50g	29.3	1	3.5	155	657
BUTTER (see also FAT AND MARGARINE)					
clarified (ghee), 1tbsp	0	0	17	150	630
garlic, 1tbsp	0	0	16.5	145	610
regular, average, 1tbsp	0	0	16.5	145	610
reduced-fat average, 1tbsp	0	0	8	76	320
CABBAGE					
chinese, raw, 40g	0	0.6	0	3	14
chinese, flowering (pak choi), raw, 40g	0	1	0	5	20
mustard (dai gai choi), raw, 75g	0.5	2	0	11	45
red, raw, 40g	1	1.2	0	9.5	40
red, cooked, 60g	2	1	0	12	50
rolls, Lebanese, 3 small, 250g	40	+	10	290	1220
savoy, cooked, 60g	1	1.5	0	10	40
savoy, raw, 40g	1	1.5	0	7	30
CAKE					
angel, average slice	40.5	N	0.5	181	760
apricot crumble tea cake, 100g	44	+	15	324	1360
apple, average slice	40	+	10	252	1060
banana cake, 100g	68	+	16	428	1800
banana madeira, 100g	58	+	13.5	367	1540
banana tea loaf, 100g	57	+	12	351	1475
battenburg, 100g	50	N	17.5	370	1551
Bavarian chocolate, 100g	30	N	22.5	332	1395
black forest, 100g	40	N	17	331	1390
bran loaf, large slice, 100g	58.4	4.6	1.6	254	1081
cake mix, sponge, made up, 50g	27	N	8	280	1220
carrot cake, bought, 100g	44	+	23	402	1690
carrot cake, fingers, 100g	64	+	17	420	1770
cheesecake, 100g	30	0.4	20	320	1350
cherry cake, 100g	61.7	1.1	15.8	384	1657
chinese cakes, 100g	51.9	N	21.5	415	1740
chocolate, 100g	55	N	17	391	1645
christmas, 1 piece, 60g	33.5	+	6	193	810
coconut, 100g	51.2	2.5	23.8	434	1815
crispie cakes, 100g	73.1	0.3	18.6	464	1951
date loaf, 1 piece, 55g	27	+	4.5	158	665

BUTTER & MARGARINE Which

is healthier? In fact, they both have the same fat and calorie content, though margarines are usually lower in saturated fat than butter. Replacing butter, for example, with a polyunsaturated fat or monounsaturated spread may help reduce cholesterol levels in the blood. However, try to use all spreads sparingly.

BUTTER By law, butter must contain over 80% fat. This fat is predominantly saturated and high in cholesterol.

DAIRY SPREADS Gaining in popularity, these spreads have some canola or olive oil added but they can still contain up to 42% saturated fat.

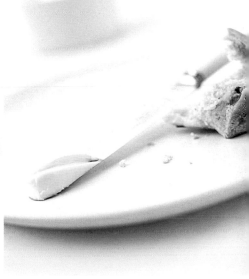

POLYUNSATURATED MARGARINES These are usually made with sunflower, safflower and soya bean oils. Replacing saturates in the diet with polyunsaturates may help lower blood cholesterol levels. Some margarines that are high in polyunsaturates are now available in reduced-fat varieties.

REDUCED-FAT SPREADS A blend of milk fat or vegetable oil and water, with about 50% of the fat of butter or margarine.

FOOD	CARB	FIBRE	FAT	ENERGY	
	g	g	g	kcal	kJ
CAKE CONT.					
date & walnut loaf, 1 piece, 60g	32	+	6	189	795
eclair, chocolate, bought, 70g	22.5	0.5	18	264	1110
flan, fruit, 100g	28.5	0.7	8	187	785
fruit, plain, 1 piece, 50g	271	+	6	165	695
fruit, retail, 1 piece, 70g	39	0.7	7	225	945
fruit cake, iced, 70g	43.9	1.2	8	249	1053
fruit cake, rich, 1 slice, 70g	41.7	1.2	7.7	239	1007
gateau, 1 slice, 85g	36.9	0.3	143	286	1201
gingerbread, 50g	32.4	0.6	6.3	190	800
hazelnut torte, average slice	N	+	30	402	1690
jam fairy, 100g	58.5	N	18	417	1750
jam sponge, 100g	67.5	1.8	2.5	312	1310
lamington, bought, 1, 75g	36	+	9	233	980
lamington, cream-filled, 1, 60g	30	+	7	187	785
lemon rolls, 100g	60.5	N	15	360	1510
madeira, 1 slice, 40g	23.4	0.4	6.8	157	661
madeira, iced, 100g	58	N	14	369	1550
marble, 100g	60	N	13.5	374	1570
mud, 100g	59	N	20	428	1800
rock, 1 medium, 60g	33	0.8	8	221	930
rum baba, average serving	47	N	10	326	1370
sponge cake, average slice, 60g	31.4	0.5	15.8	275	1152
sponge cake, fatless, 1 slice, 58g	30.7	0.5	3.5	171	722
sponge, fairy, 100g	60.5	N	8.5	344	1445
sponge, jam-filled, 1 slice, 60g	38.5	1.1	2.9	181	768
sponge with butter icing, slice, 60g	31.4	0.4	18.4	294	1228
swiss roll, 1 slice, 35g	22.5	0.5	2.5	114	480
swiss roll, chocolate, individual, 25g	14.5	N	2.8	84	355
CAPERS					
1 tbsp	1	+	0	7	30
CAPSICUM					
green, raw, 100g	2.5	1.6	0	15	65
red, raw, 100g	4	1.6	0	25	105
CAROB					
bar, 1, 45g	18	+	11.5	186	780
coated biscuit 1, 18g	9.5	N	5.5	89	375
powder, 2 tbsp, 40g	15	+	0	59	250
CARROT					
baby, raw, peeled, 50g	3	1.2	0	13	55
canned, 100g	4	1.9	0,	20	85
juice, 125ml	8	+	0	39	165
raw, peeled, boiled, 70g	4	2	0	19	80
CASSAVA peeled, boiled, 100g	30.5	1.6	0.5	131	550
CAULIFLOWER					
boiled, 100g	2	1.6	0	19	80
cheese, 200g	11	2	20	269	1130
raw, 50g	1	1	0	9	40

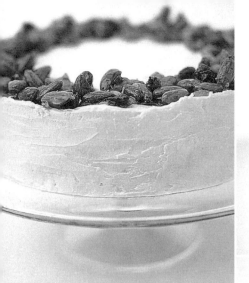

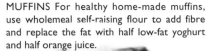

MUFFINS For healthy home-made muffins, use wholemeal self-raising flour to add fibre and replace the fat with half low-fat yoghurt and half orange juice.

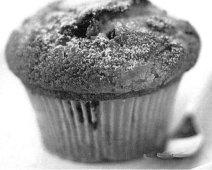

CARROT CAKE Long thought to be a 'healthy cake', it can in fact contain up to a cup of oil. The cream cheese icing is high in fat and sugar.

RECIPE Fat-free sponge cake can be made by combining eggs, sugar, plain flour and baking powder. Add decoration and flavour with some high-fibre, sliced fruit.

CAKE As a general rule, the lighter and whiter the cake, the lower its fat content. Small amounts of any cake, as an occasional treat, can be eaten as part of a healthy diet. However, as a healthier option, go for fat-free sponge (see recipe) and fruit cakes (which contain more fibre) than creamy cakes with jam or butter icing. For increased fibre content, try making cakes with wholemeal flour.

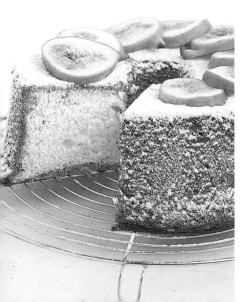

SWISS ROLL A jam filling is less fattening than a cream one, though jam will increase the sugar content.

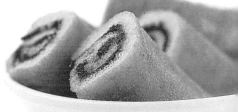

FOOD	CARB g	FIBRE g	FAT g	ENERGY kcal	kJ
CELERIAC					
fresh, Peeled, boiled, 100g	5.5	3.2	0	31	130
fresh, peeled, 120g	5	4.5	0	29	120
CELERY					
chopped, boiled, 63g	1.5	0.7	0	8	35
raw, 2 x 10cm sticks, 40g	1	0.5	0.5	5	20
CEREAL					
bran strands, 40g	18.6	9.8	1.4	104	444
bran with fruit and oats, 45g	34.5	9	1.5	138	580
bran, natural, 12g	7.5	4.5	0.5	33	140
bran, oat, unprocessed, 2 tbsp, 22g	11	3.5	1.5	53	225
bran, rice, 15g	7.5	4	3	70	295
bran, wheat, processed, 45g	31	14	2.5	161	675
bran, wheat, unprocessed, 2 tbsp, 10g	1	4	0.5	15	65
branflakes, 30g	20.8	3.9	0.6	95	406
chocolate flavoured rice pops, 30g	28.3	0.2	0.3	115	491
cornflakes, 30g	25.8	0.3	0.2	108	461
cornflakes, with nuts, 30g	26.6	0.2	1.2	119	507
crispies, rice based, 30g	27	0.2	0.3	111	472
crunchy oat bran flakes with fruit, 45g	31	N	2	160	675
crunchy oat bran flakes, 30g	22.2	3	1.2	107	456
fruit & fibre flakes, 30g	21.6	2.1	1.4	105	444
fruit & nut wheat flakes, 45g	31	3	1.5	157	660
grapenuts, 30g	25.5	+	1	113	475
high-energy multi flakes, 100g	81.7	2	1.7	355	1504
high-energy wheat flakes, 45g	35.5	2	1.5	170	715
high-protein rice flakes, 30g	24.5	0.6	0.3	113	481
honeynut cornflakes, 30g	26.6	0.2	1.2	119	507
honey wheat puffs, 30g	26.6	0.9	0.6	116	493
instant oats, 36g	24.7	2.6	2.8	134	569
muesli, swiss style, 50g	36.1	3.2	3	182	770
muesli with no added sugar, 50g	33.5	3.8	3.9	183	776
muesli, apricot & almond, 60g	35.5	+	4.5	210	880
muesli, apricot toasted, 30g	20	+	3	121	510
muesli, natural, 60g	39.5	2	2.5	208	875
muesli, oat & honey, 45g	31	+	7	188	790
muesli, traditional, 60g	37	2	4	221	930
muesli flakes, 45g	32	+	1	157	660
multigrain flakes, 30g	21.5	1	3	115	485
nut crunchie clusters, 45g	33.5	+	3.5	177	745
oat bran, crunchy, 45g	30	+	2.5	170	710
oat bran & fruit, 40g	30.5	+	3.5	168	705
oat bran, 30g	23.5	+	1.5	115	485
porridge oats made with water, 200g	18	1.6	2.2	98	418
porridge, made with whole milk, 200g	27.4	1.6	10.2	232	976
puffed wheat, 20g	13.5	1.1	0.3	64	273
puffed wheat with honey, 30g	25.4	1	0.2	104	445
puffed wheat, sugar coated, 30g	25.4	1	0.2	104	445

CEREAL BRANS

CEREAL BRANS Eating a healthy diet with plenty of fibre may help to prevent cancer of the bowel and constipation, and cereal brans (the husks of grain) are a concentrated source. However, uncooked bran contains phytates that hinder the absorption of minerals. The best way to boost your fibre intake is with wholegrain cereals and breads, legumes, fruit and vegetables.

HIGH-FIBRE BREAKFAST Packed with fibre, baked beans on a piece of wholemeal toast or muffin is a great start to the day.

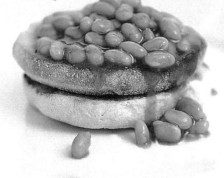

RECIPE Make a high-fibre smoothie by blending low-fat soya milk, yoghurt, a banana, honey and a tablespoon of oat bran.

BRAN CEREALS Processed bran cereals are a good, high-fibre alternative to raw bran, but check the labels for added salt and sugar.

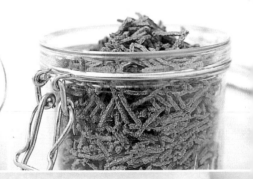

HOW MUCH? A tablespoon of bran provides a sixth of the recommended 30g of fibre a day. This is similar to the amount of fibre in a slice of wholemeal bread.

FOOD	CARB	FIBRE	FAT	ENERGY	
	g	g	g	kcal	kJ
CEREAL CONT.					
rice puffs, 30g	26.9	0.2	0.3	111	472
rice puffs, sugar coated, 30g	28.7	0.1	0.2	114	487
small whole wheat biscuits, 45g	33.3	4.3	0.7	149	635
small whole wheat biscuits with added fruit, 40g	30.2	3.2	0.8	135	573
sugar coated cornflakes, 30g	28.1	0.2	0.2	113	482
sultana bran flakes, 50g	34	5	0.8	150	645
wheat biscuits, 1, 20g	15	1.9	0.5	70	300
wheat flakes, 30g	24	2.6	0.8	108	459
wheat flakes and raisins, 40g	26	4	1.5	140	585
wheat rings, 100g	86.1	N	2.7	372	1581
wheat biscuits, 2, 40g	30	3.8	1	140	600
whole wheat biscuit, 1, 22g	15	2.2	0.7	72	304
CEREAL BAR (see also MUESLI BAR)					
apricot fruity bar, 1 small	18	+	2.5	105	440
low sugar, 1 large	26	+	2.5	136	570
sports, 1	28.5	+	2.5	145	610
CHEESE					
blue brie, 30g	0	0	13.5	126	530
blue castello, 30g	0	0	10	110	465
blue vein, 30g	0	0	9.5	110	465
bocconcini, 20g	0	0	7	76	320
brie, 30g	0	0	8.5	101	425
camembert, 30g	0	0	8	92	385
canola, mild, 30g	0	0	6.5	94	395
cheddar, 30g	0	0	10	122	505
cheddar, low-fat, 30g	0	0	7	99	410
cheddar, processed, 30g	0	0	8	99	415
cheddar, reduced-fat, 30g	0	0	7	98	410
cheddar slices, 20g	1	0	4.5	61	255
cheddar slices, reduced-fat, 20g	1	0	3	48	200
cheddar sticks, 20g	1	0	6	67	280
cheshire, 30g	0	0	10	114	480
cottage, 1tbsp	0	0	2	29	120
cottage, with cheese, 1tbsp	0.5	0	0.5	17	70
cottage, low-fat, 1tbsp	0.5	0	0.5	18	75
cottage with pineapple, low-fat, 1tbsp	3	0.5	0	27	115
creamed cottage, 1tbsp	0.5	0	1	24	100
creamed cottage, low-fat, 1tbsp	1	0	0.5	19	80
cream, 30g	1	0	10	101	425
cream, fruit, 30g	0	0	7.5	83	350
cream, light, 30g	1	0	5	48	200
cream, full fat, 30g	0.5	0	10	102	430
double Gloucester, 30g	0	0	10	120	505
edam, 30g	0	0	8	106	445
emmental, 30g	0	0	9	113	475
fetta, 30g	0	0	7	83	350
goat's, 30g	0.5	0	4.5	58	245

MUESLI This usually contains wheat and oat flakes with nuts and dried fruit. Choose varieties with no 'added' sugar. Muesli is high in fibre and a good source of many vitamins and minerals.

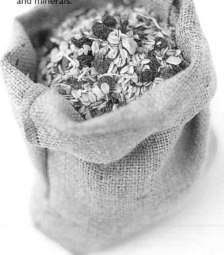

RECIPE If you love toasted muesli, try this low-fat version. Combine 2½ cups rolled oats, ½ cup oat bran and 175g mixed dried fruit and seeds. Drizzle with a very small amount of maple syrup and bake in a 180°C/350°F (Gas 4) oven for 20 minutes.

CEREAL Starchy foods such as breakfast cereals are an important part of a healthy diet. They provide carbohydrates, fibre and are often fortified with vitamins and minerals. However, it's best to avoid 'frosted' cereals or those containing 'added' sugar. Some cereals may also be high in fat and salt. Always check the label and try to choose wholegrain varieties.

SPORTS CEREALS Advertised as being the ideal way to begin your day, a lot of these are high in sugar, though relatively low in fat.

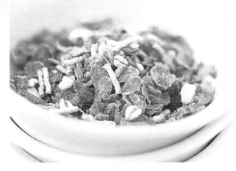

WHEAT BISCUITS These, together with other wholewheat cereals, are usually sugar free, low in fat and high in fibre. They make an excellent, filling start to the day.

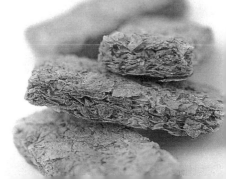

FOOD	CARB g	FIBRE g	FAT g	ENERGY kcal	kJ
CHEESE CONT.					
gouda, 30g	0	0	9	113	475
halloumi, 30g	0	0	5	73	305
havarti, 30g	0	0	11	120	505
jarisberg, 30g	0	0	9	113	475
jarlsberg lite, 30g	0	0	5	82	346
lancashire, 30g	0	0	9.5	110	465
leicester, 30g	0	0	10	119	500
mozzarella, 30g	0	0	6.5	90	380
mozzarella, reduced-fat, 30g	0	0	5.5	86	360
parmesan, 30g	0	0	9.5	132	555
pizza, grated, 30g	0	0	6.5	93	390
processed, 30g	0	0	7	42	175
quark, 20g	0	0	2.5	26	110
quark, low-fat, 20g	0	0	0.5	15	65
reduced-fat, 20g	0	0	4.5	69	290
ricotta, 20g	0	0	2	30	125
ricotta, reduced-fat, 20g	0.5	0	1.5	25	105
ricotta, smooth, 20g	0	0	2	25	105
sheep's milk, fresh, 30g	0	0	6.5	90	380
soft, 30g	0	0	10	124	520
soya, 30g	0	0	8	93	390
stilton, 30g	0	0	9.5	111	465
swiss, 30g	0	0	9	114	480
wensleydale, 30g	0	0	9.5	112	470
CHERRIES					
canned in syrup, drained, 100g	17	0.6	0	70	295
glace, 6, 30g	20	0.3	0	77	325
raw, weighed with stones, 100g	12	0.7	0.1	53	225
CHEWING GUM					
sugarless, per piece, 10g	0	0	0	4	15
with sugar, per piece, 10g	3	0	0	9.5	40
CHICKEN					
breast, no skin, grilled, 100g	0	0	5	157	660
breast, with skin, grilled, 100g	0	0	12.5	218	915
breast, quarter, no skin, barbecued, 100g	0	0	6	199	835
breast, quarter, with skin, rotisseried, 100g	N	0	12.5	214	900
breast, lean, 100g	0	0	1	40	170
chicken pastrami, 1 serving, 30g	N	N	1	40	170
crispy-skinned, 100g	0	0	3	64	270
drumstick, no skin, baked, 2	0	0	9	179	750
drumstick, with skin, baked, 2	0	0	14.5	229	960
drumstick crumbed, 145g	N	0	17	313	1315
fried chicken (see FAST FOOD)					
nuggets, 1, 20g	2.5	0	3.5	57	240

CHEESE Belonging in the milk and dairy food section of the food wheel (see page 6), cheese should be consumed in moderation. It is an excellent source of calcium — the mineral essential for healthy teeth and bones. Many cheeses are relatively high in fat, although reduced-fat varieties are becoming increasingly available.

PARMESAN Hard cheeses can contain up to 35% fat, but with parmesan, the strong flavour means that, though high in fat, a little can go a long way. Grate with the fine side of the grater and you'll end up using less cheese.

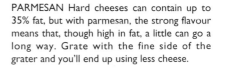

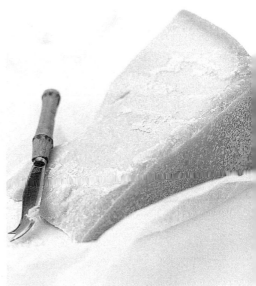

COTTAGE CHEESE The winner in the low-fat competition. Buy the low-fat version and use as a spread, for dips or as a sandwich filling.

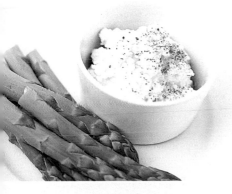

MOZZARELLA Pizza-lovers take note, this cheese is relatively high in fat (about 21%). If you're making pizza at home, replace half with low fat mozzarella, so you get lots of taste, but less fat.

RICOTTA On average, this contains about 11% fat, compared to hard cheeses such as cheddar, which contain about 35% fat. However, although it is relatively low in fat, it is often used in popular Italian desserts, which aren't so healthy!

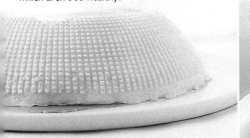

FOOD	CARB	FIBRE	FAT	ENERGY	
	g	g	g	kcal	kJ
CHICKEN CONT.					
roll, processed, 1 slice, 38g	4.5	N	9.5	158	665
sausage, cooked, skinless, 2	0	0	10	164	690
thigh, no skin, cooked, 2	0	0	6	126	530
thigh, with skin, cooked, 2	0	0	8	145	610
wing, with skin, cooked, 2	0	0	12	179	750
CHICKPEAS					
canned, drained, 186g	29.9	7.6	5.4	214	906
dried, boiled, 180g	32.8	7.7	3.8	218	922
CHICORY GREENS					
raw, 100g	2.8	1	0.6	11	45
CHILLI					
powder, 1 tsp, 5g	Tr	Tr	0	N	N
green, raw, each, 20g	1	N	0	4	15
red, raw, each, 20g	1	0.3	0	6	25
CHIVES					
fresh, 2 tbsp, 40g	Tr	0.8	0	1	5
CHOCOLATE					
after-dinner mint, 1, 6g	11	0	1.5	87	365
block, 100g	55.5	N	32.5	536	2250
coconut, bar, 1, 57g	33.2	+	14.9	270	1129
caramels, 1, 20g	12	0	5.5	99	415
cherry-flavoured centre, 1, 55g	30.5	0	13.5	248	1040
cream, 100g	43	N	46.5	604	2535
cooking, dark, 100g	56	+	31	505	2120
cooking, milk, 100g	61.5	+	28.5	505	2120
coated waffer biscuits, 1, 45g	27	N	11.5	220	945
coated candies, 1 packet, 55g	40	N	10.5	257	1080
coated peanuts, 1 packet, 55g	34	+	13.5	273	1145
coated malt balls, 1 packet, 45g	30	N	9.5	212	890
coated nougat and toffee bar, 1, medium, 65g	43.2	+	12.3	285	1204
coated nougat bar, 1, 25g	13.5	N	9	137	575
coated whipped bar, 1, 26g	16.5	+	4.1	103	435
coated biscuit fruit and nut bar, 1, 55g	27.5	+	16.5	280	1175
coated peanut bar, 1, 60g	36	+	13.5	283	1190
coated biscuit, 1, 55g	35	+	13.8	264	1128
choc bar, 1, 40g	23	+	11.5	204	855
full cream, milk, 1, 54g	32.1	+	16.4	286	1196
fruit & nut bar, 100g	54	+	34	540	2270
honeycomb bar, 80g	56	0	163	387	1625
in crisp sugar shells, 1 tube, 37g	27.3	+	6.5	169	711
soft centres, 100g	64.5	0	21.5	469	1970

BBQ CHICKEN Better than deep-fried chicken because fat is lost during cooking on the rotisserie. Avoid the skin, as that is where the fat is hidden.

CHICKEN A good source of protein and B vitamins. If you are watching the amount of fat in your diet, avoid the skin of the chicken, which makes up about 50% of its fat content (remove it before cooking if possible). Without its skin, chicken is a low-fat source of protein, especially if you poach, steam or grill it.

RECIPE For a low-fat dinner, brush a skinless chicken breast or thigh fillet with a mixture of sweet chilli sauce, soy sauce and chopped fresh coriander. Barbecue or grill.

ROAST CHICKEN The juices that come out of a roasting chicken are high in saturated fat. Instead, place on a rack inside a pan and baste with a little oil.

BREASTS VS THIGHS Although chicken breast can be 2 or 3g lower in fat than the same amount of thigh meat, it tends to dry out if cooked for too long. Thighs are perfect for slower cooking in curries and casseroles.

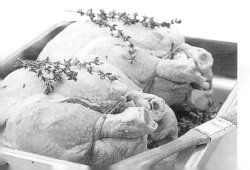

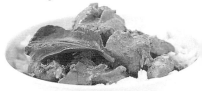

FOOD	CARB	FIBRE	FAT	ENERGY	
	g	g	g	kcal	kJ
CHOCOLATE CONT.					
triangular nougat bar, 1, 50g	28.5	N	15	264	1110
CHUTNEY					
fruit, homemade, 1 tbsp	8.5	0.4	0	34	145
mango, 1 tbsp	9	0.2	0	30	125
COCOA POWDER					
1 tbsp	1.5	1.2	1	21	90
COCONUT					
cream, block, 100g	7	+	68.8	669	2760
desiccated, dried, 25g	1.6	3.4	15.5	151	623
oil, 1 tbsp	0	0	20	176	740
COFFEE					
for each teaspoon of sugar in coffee, add ...	5	0	0	19	80
cappuccino, whole milk, 1 cup, 200ml	N	0	5	89	375
cappuccino, skim milk, 1 cup, 200ml	N	0	0	50	210
decaffeinated, black, 1 cup, 200ml	0	0	0	0	0
filtered, black, 1 cup, 200ml	Tr	0	0	7	30
ground, 1 cup + 25ml whole milk, 225ml	2.5	0	1	23	95
ground, 1 cup + 25ml skim milk, 225ml	2.5	0	0	18	75
iced, plain, 1 cup, 200ml	1.5	0	7	59	250
iced, with whole milk ice cream					
& cream, 325 ml	N	0	12	179	750
instant black, 1 cup, 200ml	0	0	0	2	8
instant, 1 cup + 25ml whole milk, 225ml	1.5	0	1	18	75
instant, 1 cup + 25ml skim milk, 225ml	1.5	0	0	13	55
Irish, 1 cup, 200ml	Tr	0	10	189	795
milk, 1 tsp coffee + 1 cup whole milk, 200ml	12.5	0	10	173	725
mocha, 1 cup, 200ml	N	0	10	119	500
percolated, black, 1, cup, 200ml	Tr	0	0	0	0
whitener, 1 tsp	2	0	1.5	21	90
CORDIAL (see also SOFT DRINKS)					
citrus, 25% juice, prepared, 1 glass, 250ml	17	0	0	65	275
citrus, 60% juice, prepared, 1 glass, 250ml	18	0	0	73	.305
citrus, reduced sugar					
lemon, prepared, 1 glass, 250ml	N	0	0	69	290
undiluted, 1 tbsp	9	0	0	34	145
CORN					
baby, canned, 6, 100g	2	1.5	0.4	23	96
cob, 1, large, 100g	11.6	1.3	1.4	66	280
creamed, canned, 100g	20	+	1	81	340
kernels, canned, 30g	8	0.4	0.4	37	156
CORN CHIPS (see also SNACK FOOD)					
cheese, 40g	25.5	2	9.5	193	810
flavoured, 40g	20	2	12	198	830
toasted snacks, 40g	21.7	0.4	12.8	208	867
CORNMEAL dry, 40g	30	1	0.5	145	610
COUSCOUS cooked, 100g	23	+	0	112	470
CRABAPPLE raw, 60g	12	+	0	45	190

MILK CHOCOLATE This is usually made by adding milk solids to chocolate. It has the same sugar content as dark and white chocolate.

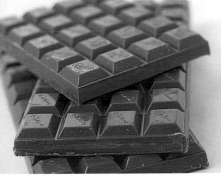

CHOCOLATE Good for an occasional energy boost, a chocolate bar is, however, high in fat and sugar and does contain caffeine. Chocolate is made up of about 30% fat, usually in the form of cocoa butter, and this is what gives chocolate its melt-in-the-mouth texture. Carob is also high in fat, although it is caffeine-free.

WHITE CHOCOLATE Not a true chocolate because it doesn't contain cocoa solids. It is, however, still made from cocoa butter, milk and sugar, and is high in fat.

DARK CHOCOLATE All chocolate is high in fat. However, high-quality chocolate has less sugar and, where this is the case, cocoa solids will come before sugar in the ingredients. Good-quality bitter chocolate has the least sugar.

COCOA The process of manufacturing cocoa powder removes much of the fat content (cocoa butter). Use in cooking to add chocolate flavour without too much fat.

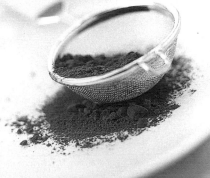

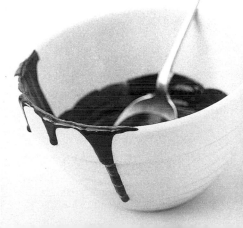

FOOD	CARB	FIBRE	FAT	ENERGY	
	g	g	g	kcal	kJ
CRACKERS (see also CRISPBREAD)					
cheese flavour, 2	4	+	1	24	100
cream, 2	4.5	0.4	2	40	170
rye, 2	5.5	1.6	1.5	38	160
rice snacks, cheese, 30g	22	+	2	117	490
rice snacks, sesame, 30g	22	+	2	117	490
sesame, 2	3	+	1	20	85
water crackers, 2	4.5	0.4	0.5	25	105
CRANBERRY JUICE 1 glass, 250ml	36.5	N	0	143	600
CREAM					
aerosol, whipped, 100ml	4	0	30.5	293	1230
clotted, 100ml	2	0	63	586	2413
crème fraîche, 100ml	2.5	0	48	440	1850
double thick, rich, 100ml	3	0	54.5	499	2095
light, 100ml	3.5	0	17.5	189	795
regular, 100ml	3	0	35.5	333	1400
thickened, 100ml	3.5	0	36.5	345	1450
thickened, light, 100ml	6	0	19	211	885
CREAM, SOUR					
extra light, 100ml	7	0	12.5	158	665
light, 100ml	5	0	18	193	810
regular, dairy 100ml	4	0	19	199	835
CREPE plain, 20g	7.5	0.5	2.5	65	275
CRISPBREAD					
high fibre, 1, 5g	4	1	0	17	70
bran & malt, 1	3.5	0.5	0	19	80
plain, 1	4.5	0.5	1	27	115
rye, 1, 10g	7.1	1.2	0.2	32	137
fat-free, 1	7	+	0	34	145
original, low fat, 1	5	+	1	32	135
puffed, 1	4	N	0	19	80
wholemeal, 1	5	+	1	29	120
swiss type, 1	16	1.2	0.5	79	330
− with sesame whole rye, 1	15	1.2	1	81	340
− multigrain, 1	9	1.2	1.5	60	250
− wholemeal, 1	9	1	1	58	245
wheatgerm type, original, 1	4	1	0.5	23	95
CROISSANT plain, 60g	23	1	12.2	216	903
CROUTONS 1 serving, 15g	11	1	1	61	255
CRUMPET					
regular, toasted, 40g	17.4	0.8	0.4	80	338
wholemeal, toasted, 45g	17	1.5	0.5	85	355
CUCUMBER					
lebanese, raw, unpeeled, 5 slices, 35g	1	0.5	0	4	15
raw, unpeeled, 5 slices, 45g	3	0.5	0	4	15
CUMQUAT (KUMQUAT)					
raw, peeled, 1, 20g	3	0.8	0	12	50
CURRANTS dried, 75g	50.9	1.4	0.3	200	854

RECIPE For a delicious low-fat alternative to cream, try combining low-fat ricotta with a little low-fat vanilla yoghurt.

IMITATION CREAMS These are not necessarily lower in fat than 'real' creams, but the saturated fat content tends to be lower because they are often made with vegetable rather than milk fats.

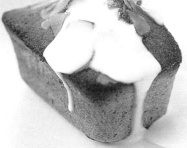

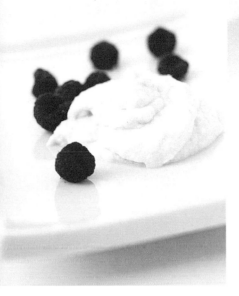

CREAM A concentrated source of saturated fat and calories. However, not all creams have the same fat content; a general rule is the thicker the cream, the higher the fat content. For example, single cream contains about 19% fat whereas clotted cream contains about 63% fat! Consider using low-fat yoghurt as a dessert alternative.

HALF-FAT CREAM This has about 13% fat – half that of full cream. However, if you use low-fat yoghurt as a substitute, you will reduce the fat level to just 1%.

EXTRA THICK CREAM Containing about 54% fat, this cream is a thick, rich and very indulgent treat

FOOD	CARB	FIBRE	FAT	ENERGY	
	g	g	g	kcal	kJ
CURRY PASTE					
curry paste, 1tbsp	1.5	N	2	24	100
curry powder 1tbsp	3	2.8	1.5	30	125
hot curry paste, 1tbsp	1.5	N	2	26	110
Indian, 1tbsp	5	0	9	98	410
tandoori, 1tbsp	2	0	0	49	205
CUSTARD					
baked, egg, 100ml	9	0	4.5	95	400
bread & butter custard, 100ml	15.5	0.5	5.5	132	555
custard & fruit, 100ml	16	+	1.5	86	360
powder, prepared with whole milk, 100ml	12.5	0	4	96	405
powder, prepared with reduced-fat milk 100ml	13.5	0	1.5	82	345
pouring, regular, 100ml	16	0	1.5	88	370
DANISH PASTRY					
almond, 100g	46	2	25	428	1800
apple, 100g	43.5	N	12	298	1250
apricot, 100g	38	N	12	270	1135
blueberry, 100g	40	N	12	286	1200
chocolate, 100g	24	N	19.5	280	1175
continental,100g	37.5	N	17	325	1365
custard, 100g	34.5	N	17	307	1290
pecan, 100g	52	N	20.5	417	1750
DATES					
dried, 6, 50g	28.5	2	0	113	485
fresh, seeded, chopped, 50g	14.5	0.9	0	54	228
DESSERT					
apple pie, bakery, 100g	28	+	8.5	198	830
apple pie, manufatured, 100g	38.5	1.7	12.5	279	1170
apple pie, reduced fat, 100g	32.5	+	7	199	835
apple & blackberry pie, 100g	42.5	+	17	336	1410
apple & rhubarb crumble, 120g	44	2	8	250	1050
apple strudel, 100g	41	+	11	273	1145
apricot pie, 100g	33	+	10	232	975
apricot pie, bought, 100g	38.5	+	14	293	1230
banana split with 3 scoops ice cream	55	1.1	10.5	325	1365
chocolate mocha, 100g	32.5	N	23.5	349	1465
bavarian, chocolate swirl, 100g	30.5	0	19.5	306	1285
blackberry & apple pie, 100g	35	+	10	232	975
chocolate mousse, 100g	28	0	13	232	975
chocolate mousse, dessert, 100g	23	0	9	201	845
chocolate mousse, light, 100g	19	0	4	136	570
Christmas pudding, 1 piece, 50g	29	1	6	167	700
custard tart 1, 135g	41	1.5	17.5	350	1470
junket (blancmange), 100g	48	0	3.5	114	480
lemon meringue pie, 1 piece, 75g	28.5	0.5	12.5	238	1000
pecan pie, 1 piece, 115g	64.5	+	21	450	1890
profiteroles, 1, 55g	N	+	9	130	545
pudding, blackberry sponge, 100g	59.9	+	5	299	1255

BACK-TO-BASICS Home-made rice custard or bread-and-butter pudding made with skimmed milk are great reduced fat desserts.

PIES AND TARTS The pastry in these tend to make them a high-fat option. Save them for occasional treats and choose fruit-based ones where possible.

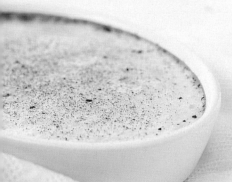

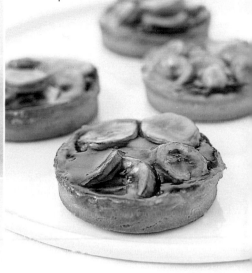

DESSERT

A sweet treat is a perfect way to end a meal, and it doesn't have to be high in fat. A fruit sorbet is a delicious dessert with no fat at all, while pancakes or puddings made with low-fat dairy products are full of energy-giving carbohydrates. Fruit, eaten on its own or with some low-fat yoghurt, is one of the tastiest and healthiest desserts of all.

RECIPE Bring 1 cup of low-calorie cordial, 4 cups of water and a cinnamon stick to the boil. Add a peeled pear and simmer for 10–15 minutes until tender. Serve with low fat fromage frais.

CANNED FRUITS Fruits cooked in their own juice rather than in a sugar syrup are lower in calories.

FOOD	CARB	FIBRE	FAT	ENERGY	
	g	g	g	kcal	kJ
DESSERTS CONT.					
pudding, bread & butter, 100g	N	0.3	10	299	1255
pudding, chocolate mousse, 100g	32	N	6	209	880
pudding, chocolate sponge, 100g	41.5	+	4	217	910
pudding, creme caramel, 100g	20	N	3	119	500
pudding, lemon sponge, 100g	41	+	3	204	855
pudding, plum, 60g	30	+	4.5	164	690
pudding, rice, banana, canned, 125g	N	+	13	244	1025
pudding, rice, canned, 150g	22.5	0.3	3.75	135	562
pudding, rice, chocolate, canned, 125g	N	+	6.5	209	880
souffle, 100g	10.5	N	14.5	200	840
tiramisu, 100g	N	N	20	328	1380
trifle, bought, 120g	33	0.5	7	209	880
DEVON split, 50g	3	+	9	117	490
DIPS					
barbecue, 1tbsp	2.5	0	4.5	51	215
chicken & asparagus, 1tbsp	2	0	3	40	170
chilli, chip & dip type, 1tbsp	1.5	N	0	8	35
chive & onion, 1tbsp	1	0	6.5	65	275
chunky bean, 1tbsp	2.5	+	0	11	45
corn & bacon, 1tbsp	2	+	1	20	85
corn relish, 1tbsp	2	0	3	37	155
cucumber & yoghurt, 1tbsp	0	+	2	26	110
French onion, reduced fat, 1tbsp	1	0	3.5	43	180
French onion, average, 1tbsp	0	0	5	61	255
French onion, low-fat, 1tbsp	3	0	2.5	42	175
gherkin dip, 1tbsp	3	+	4	49	205
herb & garlic, 1tbsp	2	+	4	45	190
hot & spicy, 1tbsp	2	0	3.5	44	185
hummus, 1tbsp	2	0.6	3.5	45	190
taramasalata, 1tbsp	2	+	4	46	195
DOLMADES 60g	14.5	+	4	101	425
DOUGHNUT					
cinnamon sugar, 1 large, 75g	36.6	+	10.9	252	1061
cream-filled, 1, 70g	21	+	17	251	1055
iced, 1, 80g	38.5	+	19.5	339	1425
DRESSINGS (see also MAYONNAISE)					
caesar, 1tbsp	3	0	7	76	320
caesar, creamy, 1tbsp	2	0	7	70	295
coleslaw, average, 1tbsp	7	0	7	88	370
coleslaw, reduced fat, 1tbsp	5	0	7	82	345
coleslaw, light, 1tbsp	5.5	0	3.5	57	240
French, 1tbsp	2.5	0	4.5	49	205
French, olive oil, 1tbsp	3	0	3.5	43	180
French, low-fat, 1tbsp	3.5	0	0	14	60
Italian, 1tbsp	1.5	0	6	59	250
Italian, light, 1tbsp	2	0	3.5	40	170
Italian, low fat, 1tbsp	3.1	0	0	12	50

CREAMY DRESSING This can add lots of saturated fat to your salad. For a healthy alternative, combine low-fat yoghurt with orange juice, mustard and herbs.

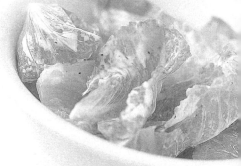

DRESSINGS

A green salad is packed with fibre, vitamins and minerals, but a heavy hand with the dressing can add lots of unwanted calories. However, the vegetable oils in most dressings contain the more healthy monounsaturated or polyunsaturated fats, as well as vitamin F. Use more juice or vinegar to oil for a zesty dressing with less fat.

VINAIGRETTE All oils have the same fat content, but extra virgin olive oil has more taste, so a little in a vinaigrette goes a long way.

RECIPE Make a low-fat juice dressing by combining orange juice, mustard, honey and a very small amount of olive oil.

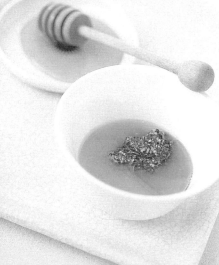

SIMPLE DRESSING Avocados contain quite a lot of fat. Instead of an oily dressing, try just a squeeze of lemon juice and some black pepper.

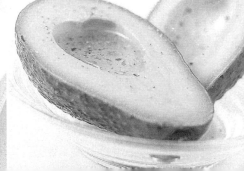

FOOD	CARB	FIBRE	FAT	ENERGY	
	g	g	g	kcal	kJ
DRESSINGS CONT.					
lemon pepper, reduced fat, 1tbsp	5	0	2	37	155
potato salad, 1tbsp	2.5	0	7	76	320
thousand island, 1tbsp	3.5	0	7	76	320
thousand island, light, 1tbsp	3.5	0	4	51	215
DRINKING POWDER					
barley type milk drink, 1tbsp	6	N	0	31	130
bournvita, 1tbsp	1.5	N	0	24	100
cocoa, 1tbsp	1.5	1.2	1	21	90
diet hot chocolate mix, 1 sachet	7	N	1	44	185
malted milk drink, 1tbsp	8	Tr	0	38	160
milk, 1tbsp	5.5	0	0.5	32	135
milkshake, strawberry, 1tbsp	12	0	0	50	210
Swiss style diet hot chocolate mix, 1 sachet	4	N	0	20	85
DUCK					
roast, no skin, 100g	0	0	9.5	182	765
roast, skin, 100g	0	0	26	307	1290
EGG					
1 small, 45g	0	0	4.5	64	270
1 medium, 55g	0	0	5.5	77	325
1 large, 60g	0	0	6	84	355
boiled 1, 53g	0	0	5.5	80	335
duck, boiled, 1, 65g	Tr	0	9	114	480
eggs benedict, 2 eggs	0	N	52	690	2900
fried, 1, 60g	0	0	8	98	410
fried, 2 × 60g, with 1 lean grilled bacon rasher	Tr	0	19	251	1055
omelette, plain or herb, 2 × 60g eggs	0	0	17	214	900
poached, 1, 60g	0	0	6	76	320
poached, 2 × 60g, with lean grilled bacon rasher	Tr	0	16	236	990
quail, raw, 1, 10g	0	0	1	15	65
replacer, 1tsp	1.5	0	1	31	130
scrambled, 2 × 60g	Tr	0	16	195	820
turkey, raw, 1, 80g	Tr	0	9.5	134	565
white only, 1, 31g	0	0	0	14	60
yolk only, 1	0	0	5	54	225
EGGPLANT (see also AUBERGINE)					
baby, 4, 65g	1.5	1.5	0	11	45
fried in oil, 100g	2.8	2.3	32	302	1262
grilled, 3 slices, 90g	2.5	2	0	18	75
raw, 100g	2.2	2	0.4	15	64
ELDERBERRIES raw, 145g	10.5	++	0.5	51	215
ENDIVE					
Belgian, raw, 60g	0	1.2	0	6	25
curly, 80g	0	1.6	0	6	25
FALAFEL commercial, 2, 60g	10	+	9	140	590
FAST FOOD (SHOP BOUGHT)					
apple pie, 1, 80g	30.5	1.3	13	239	1005
bacon & cheese chicken fillet burger, 190g	34.5	+	22.2	460	1930

EGG A good source of protein, vitamins and minerals, eggs have had a hard time because of fears about their high cholesterol level. In fact, to keep your blood cholesterol low, it is more important to avoid saturated fat in your diet. So providing they are eaten in moderation, eggs can form part of a nutritious diet.

SATURATED FAT Eggs contains about 10% fat, of which under half is saturated. The healthiest way to cook an egg is by boiling or poaching it.

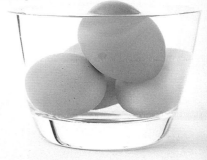

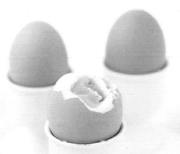

EGG YOLK Very nutritious, but also the source of cholesterol and fat in an egg.

EGG WHITE Contains no fat, so where possible, use an egg white rather than the whole egg.

RECIPE Make a reduced fat omelette by using one whole egg, 2 egg whites and some skimmed milk. Mix in fresh herbs and cook without fat in a non-stick pan.

FOOD	CARB	FIBRE	FAT	ENERGY	
	g	g	g	kcal	kJ
FAST FOOD (SHOP BOUGHT) CONT.					
bacon & cheese burger, 1, 213g	52	+	18.3	487	2045
big burger, 1, 345g	55	+	32	646	2715
chips, regular, 117g	33	2.2	20	327	1375
chips, thick cut, 95g	25	2	13	233	980
chips, thin, 110g	37.4	2.3	17	308	1291
chicken nuggets, 7, 133g	17.5	+	29.5	411	1725
chicken nuggets, 4, 76g	10	+	17	236	990
chicken fillet burger, 1, 160g	28	+	16.5	282	1185
coleslaw, small tub, 116g	16	+	7	129	540
corn, 1 cobette, 78g	17	1.1	1	89	375
cornish pastie, 1, 155g	48	1.4	31.6	515	2151
fish, battered & deep-fried, 1 fillet, 145g	20	0.6	23	365	1535
fish stick, crab-flavoured, fried, 1, 27g	3.5	0	1.5	38	160
frankfurters, boiled, 2, 100g	3.5	+	20	247	1040
french fries, small, 76g	28.5	1.5	12	226	950
french fries, regular, 114g	42.5	2.3	18	337	1415
french fries, large, 159g	59	3	25	470	1975
fried chicken, coated, 2 pieces, 154g	8.5	+	29	413	1735
grilled chicken burger, 1, 180g	43.5	+	20	484	2035
hamburger, plain, 1, 170g	38	+	17.5	379	1590
hamburger, with bacon, 1, 185g	40.5	+	24	467	1960
hamburger, with cheese, 1, 195g	41.5	+	26	501	2105
hamburger, with egg, 1, 220g	44	+	26	517	2170
hot dog, 1, 100g	18.5	+	15	246	1035
individual cheesecake, 75g	25	0.3	7	175	735
individual chocolate mousse, 75g	17	N	5.5	132	555
mashed potato & gravy, small tub, 120g	12.5	+	2	80	335
nuggets, 6 pieces, 106g	18.5	+	16.5	276	1160
sundae, caramel/chocolate, 1, 141g	36	0	9	240	1010
sundae, strawberry, 1, 141g	36	0	6.5	218	915
thickshake, average, all flavours, 1, 240g	48.5	0	8	299	1255
FAST FOOD (TAKEAWAY)					
apple pie, 1, individual, 100g	56.7	1.7	15.5	369	1554
bacon and egg muffin, 1, 145g	32.5	+	19.5	377	1585
big breakfast, 1, 250g	475	+	31	568	2385
big burger in bun, 1, 205g	40	+	30	562	2360
cheeseburger, 1, 122g	33	+	12.5	300	1260
chicken nuggets, 9 pieces, 171g	26	+	26.5	212	890
cookies, 1 box	47	+	8.5	274	1150
fillet-of-fish, 1, 146g	40	N	16	351	1475
french fries, small	37.4	2.3	17	308	1291
french fries, medium	52	3.2	22.5	414	1740
french fries, large	65	4	30	527	2215
fried chicken, 1, 184g	46	0	20.5	424	1780
hash browns, 1, 54g	15	1.5	7	124	520
hot cakes, with butter & syrup, 1 serving	85	N	15	479	2010
junior burger, 1, 100g	30	N	10	267	1120

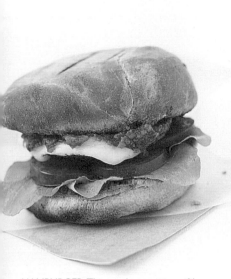

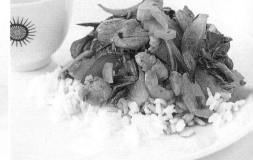

CHINESE Not too bad if you like stir-fries, but deep-fried or battered dishes are fattening. Accompany your meal with steamed rice, not fried, and note that soy sauce is high in sodium.

HAMBURGER This can be nutritious if home-made with lean mince, lettuce and tomato. If you're getting a take-away, skipping the cheese can cut the fat intake by about a third.

PIES These are generally very high in fat, especially saturated fat – even if the filling isn't meat. Try to keep your consumption of pies and pastries to a minimum.

FAST FOOD
Today, more and more people are taking advantage of take-away food. It can be high in fat but, if you look carefully, you'll find there are healthy options. A side dish of vegetables or a salad will fill you up and should be low in fat, providing it doesn't come with lashings of dressing. Choose chunky bread for sandwiches with low-fat fillings.

THAI Noodle and some stir-fried dishes are a healthy choice. Avoid curries made with coconut milk as it is high in saturated fat.

FOOD	CARB	FIBRE	FAT	ENERGY	
	g	g	g	kcal	kJ
FAST FOOD CONT.					
pan pizza, cheese, 1 slice, 105g	24.8	1.5	11.8	235	984
pan pizza, hawaiian, 1 slice, 125g	35	2	11	292	1225
pan pizza, premium range, 1 slice, 143g	35.5	2.5	15	339	1425
pan pizza, extra topping, 1 slice, 136g	32	2	16	342	1435
pizza thin crispy base, cheese, 1 slice, 79g	21.5	1.5	9	217	910
pizza thin crispy base, hawaiian, 1 slice, 99g	26	2	9.5	242	1015
pizza thin crispy base, premium type, 1 slice, 114g	25.5	2	14	289	1215
pizza thin, crispy base, extra topping, 1 slice, 114g	27	2.5	12.5	286	1200
quarter pounder burger, no cheese, 1, 176g	36	+	19.5	417	1750
sausage & egg muffin, 1, 162g	32	+	22	412	1730
sundae, hot caramel, 1, 175g	56.5	0	8	311	1305
sundae, hot fudge, 1, 175g	50	0	11	319	1340
sundae, strawberry, 1, 171g	47	Tr	6	255	1070
sundae, without topping, 1, 134g	29	0	6	183	770
samosa, meat, commercial, heated, 3, 45g	14	1	9	145	610
sausage roll, 1, 130g	31.5	1.5	23	371	1560
spring roll, deep-fried, 1 large, 175g	48	2	17	398	1670
thickshake, chocolate,					
regular, 1, 305g	60	+	9.5	360	1510
thickshake, strawberry,					
large, 1, 419g	81	0	12.5	480	2015
FAT (see also BUTTER AND FAT)					
cocoa butter, 1tbsp	0	0	20	176	740
dripping, 1tbsp	0	0	20	176	740
lard, 1tbsp	0	0	20	176	740
replacer, 1tbsp	0	0	0	75	315
shortening, 1tbsp	0	0	16	143	600
suet, 1tbsp	Tr	0	17.5	162	680
FENNEL					
raw, 1 bulb, 150g	5	3.6	0	18	75
steamed, 1 bulb, 150g	5.5	3.4	0	16	70
FIGS					
dried, 5, 75g	40	5.6	1.2	40	168
ready to eat, 30g	14	2	0.5	63	267
raw, 1, 40g	4	0.6	0	17	74
stewed, sweetened, 100g	34	3.9	0.8	143	612
FISH (see SEAFOOD)					
FLOUR					
arrowroot, 100g	94	0.1	0.1	355	1515
barley, 100g	74.5	+	1.5	344	1445
besan, chickpea, 100g	49.6	10.7	5.4	313	1328
buckwheat, 100g	76.3	2.1	1.5	364	1522
corn, 100g	92	0.1	0.7	354	1508
maize, 100g	76	+	4	363	1525
millet, 100g	75.4	N	1.7	354	1481
potato, 100g	80	5.7	0.5	329	1380
rice, 100g	80.1	2	0.8	366	1531

FISH AND CHIPS Remember that the thinner the chips, the larger the surface area, and so more fat is absorbed during frying. Try grilled fish instead of battered. Bear in mind that spring rolls, battered savs and dim sims are all high in saturated fat.

PIZZA Salami, ham and cheese are all high-fat toppings, but any pizza without cheese or meat should be a good choice. If your pizza has a filled base, that'll add calories.

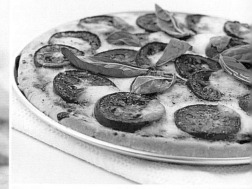

FAST FOOD

The occasional take-away meal or snack is fine if you usually eat a balanced diet. Fast food tends to be short on fresh fruit and vegetables, so a vegetarian pizza or stir-fry would be a good choice, or make up for it later in the day with a low-fat, high-fibre meal that includes an extra portion of vegetables or fruit.

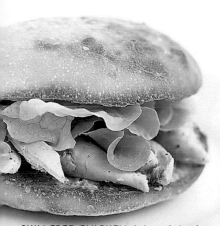

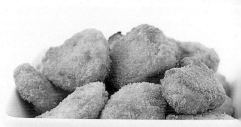

SKIN-FREE CHICKEN A lot of the fat in chicken is in the skin, so skin-free chicken is a good choice for a low-fat sandwich or burger.

CHICKEN NUGGETS For a low-fat version of these tasty snacks, cut chicken fillets into bite-size pieces, toss in egg white, then coat with cornflake crumbs. Bake in a 200°C (400°F/Gas 6) oven for 10–12 minutes.

FOOD	CARB	FIBRE	FAT	ENERGY	
	g	g	g	kcal	kJ
FLOUR CONT.					
rye, wholemeal, 100g	75.9	11.7	2	335	1428
semolina, raw, 100g	77.5	1.2	1.8	350	1489
soya, full-fat, 100g	23.5	11.2	23.5	447	1871
soya, low-fat 100g	28.2	13.5	7.2	352	1488
wheat, white, plain, 100g	77.7	3.1	1.3	341	1450
wheat, white, self-raising, 100g	75.6	3.1	1.2	330	1407
wheat, wholemeal, plain, 100g	63.9	9	2.2	310	1318
FRANKFURTER					
canned, drained, cooked, 175g	1.5	N	13	155	650
cocktail, canned. cooked, 1, 30g	0.5	0	5	62	260
cocktail, fresh, cooked, 1, 30g	1	N	6	74	310
fresh, cooked, 1, 75g	2.5	N	15	186	780
FRITTATA					
courgette & spinach, 1 slice, 250g	2	+	38.5	434	1825
Spanish (potato), 1 slice, 250g	13.5	+	27.5	369	1550
FROGS LEGS 2 fried	0	0	10	178	750
FROMAGE FRAIS					
apricot, honey & vanilla, 130g	20	0	0.5	118	495
orange tangerine, 130g	20	0	0.5	120	505
peach & mango, 130g	14.5	0	5	113	475
strawberry, 130g	15	0	5	115	485
strawberry, light, 130g	18	0	0.5	111	465
vanilla, 130g	15	0	5	115	485
vanilla, light 130g	29	0	6	230	965
petit pot, 60g	10	0	5	87	365
FROZEN DINNERS					
beef goulash, 400g	57	N	10	409	1720
beef hot-pot, 400g	39	N	11	356	1495
beef, healthy eating type, 310g	37	+	8	277	1165
bubble & squeak, 1 serving	8.5	0	2	51	215
chicken carbonara, low fat, 400g	76	N	11.5	424	1780
chicken chasseur, healthy eating type, 310g	34	+	3.5	251	1055
chicken tikka, healthy eating type, 400g	56	N	11	390	1640
curried prawns, 350g	53	N	4.6	299	1255
fettucine carbonara, 375g	49	N	30.8	552	2320
fettucine mediterranean, healthy eating type, 400g	58	N	11	395	1660
fillet of lamb, healthy eating type, 310g	9	+	8	236	990
fish fingers, grilled, 375g	15	0.5	7.5	155	650
French style chicken, low fat variety, 400g	72	N	11.5	486	2040
fried rice, 350g	20	N	7.5	390	1640
Indian style chicken, low fat, 400g	64	N	11	448	1880
roast pork, healthy eating type, 320g	34	N	5.5	277	1165
lamb, low fat, 400g	64	N	10	419	1760
shepherd's pie, 170g	13.5	1.5	8	177	745
Thai style chicken curry, low fat, 400g	64	N	12	438	1840
veal cordon bleu, healthy eating type, 320g	47	N	29	515	2165

WHITE FLOUR For those who really don't like wholemeal flour, white flour can still be nutritious and is a good protein source.

RICE FLOUR This is a good alternative to wheat flour for anyone with a gluten-intolerance. Maize cornflour, soya and potato flour are also gluten-free.

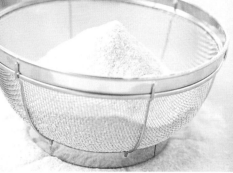

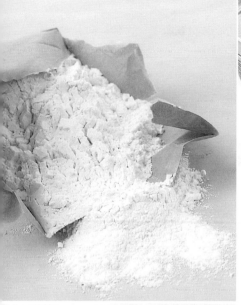

FLOUR
Made into breads, cakes, biscuits and pasta, flour is a good source of carbohydrate. Wholemeal flour is made from the whole grain, while white flour is made after the husk of the grain has been removed and, though still nutritious, does have less fibre, vitamins and minerals. Self-raising flour has more sodium than plain flour.

WHOLEMEAL Full of fibre, vitamins and minerals, wholemeal flour can be used wherever you'd use white flour in cakes, breads, biscuits and pasta-making (you may need to add a little extra water).

SOYA A strong, gluten-free flour that is a richer source of protein than most flours. It can be combined with other flours to make batters and breads.

FOOD	CARB	FIBRE	FAT	ENERGY	
	g	g	g	kcal	kJ
FRUIT (see INDIVIDUAL FRUITS)					
FRUIT BAR					
fruit fingers, apricot/strawberry/					
tropical, 1, 22g	15	1	0.5	74	310
fruit fingers, raspberry, 1 bar, 15.6g	13	+	0.5	58	245
fruit roll, 1 bar, 37.5g	23	+	2	162	680
FRUIT, DRIED (see INDIVIDUAL FRUITS)					
FRUIT SALAD (see also INDIVIDUAL FRUITS)					
canned in pear juice, drained,					
1 bowl, 220g	20.5	3.5	0	92	385
canned in syrup, drained, 1 bowl, 220g	25.5	2.5	0	106	445
fresh, 1 bowl, 140g	19.3	2.1	0.1	77	332
GARLIC					
fresh, 2 peeled cloves, 6g	0.5	+	0	6	25
powder, 1tbsp	7.5	0	0	13	55
puree, 1tbsp, 15g	2.5	N	5	57	236
GELATINE 1tbsp	0	0	0	42	175
GHERKINS drained, 36g	9	0.4	0	38	160
GINGER					
beer, dry, 1 cup, 250ml	22	0	0	82	345
gingerbread biscuit, large, figure type, 70g	34.5	1	11.5	249	1045
ground, 1tbsp	4	+	0.5	19	80
raw, peeled, grated, 1tbsp	0.5	N	0	4	15
GNOCCHI					
potato/pumpkin, average serving, 150g	13	N	12	213	895
GOLDEN SYRUP 1tbsp	21.5	0	0	83	350
GOOSE lean, roast, 100g	0	0	23	315	1325
GOOSEBERRIES					
canned, in syrup, 100g	18.5	1.7	0.2	73	310
raw, 100g	3	2.4	0	19	81
GOURD					
bottle, raw, peeled, 75g	0.6	1.9	0	8	35
ridge, raw, peeled, 75g	N	1.5	0	13	55
wax, raw, peeled, 75g	1	1	0	4	15
GRAPEFRUIT					
canned in juice, 125g	19	0.5	0	78	330
juice, sweetened, 1 glass, 200ml	19	0	0	87	365
juice, unsweetened, 1 glass, 200ml	16	0	0	71	300
raw, peeled, ½ whole, 110g	5	1	0	27	115
GRAPES					
black, 100g	15	0.7	0	63	265
black, muscatel, 100g	19	0.7	0	78	330
green, 100g	12.5	0.7	0	56	235
green, sultana, 100g	15	0.7	0	61	255
juice, sweetened, 1 glass, 200ml	N	0	1	84	355
juice, unsweetened, 1 glass, 200ml	N	0	1	84	355
GRAVY POWDER dry, 1tbsp	8	0	0.5	39	165
prepared, 225g	3	0	0	14	60

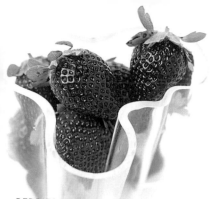

FRUIT Packed with vitamins and fibre, fruit is also low in fat and calories. According to healthy guidelines, we should all aim to eat at least five portions of fruit and vegetables every day. Choose from a variety of fresh, dried, canned (in natural juice rather than syrup) and frozen. Fruits are also rich in antioxidants (see Food Terms).

BERRIES A rich source of Vitamin C, all berries contain antioxidants and they are also low in calories.

APPLE A good source of Vitamin C and fibre, apples make a cheap, convenient, healthy snack for between meals.

PAWPAW/PAPAYA Half a medium pawpaw contains lots of beta carotene (an antioxidant) and twice the daily requirement of Vitamin C.

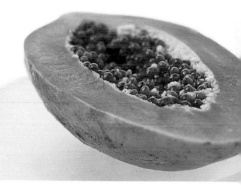

DRIED FRUITS A rich source of dietary fibre, potassium and some iron, dried fruits don't contain much vitamin C. They can also be high in 'natural' fruit sugar-fructose, which causes tooth decay in the same way as sugar.

RECIPE Place some dried fruit in a pan, cover with apple or orange juice and bring to the boil. Stand for 15 minutes until the fruit is plump, then serve warm with low-fat yoghurt.

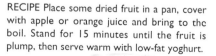

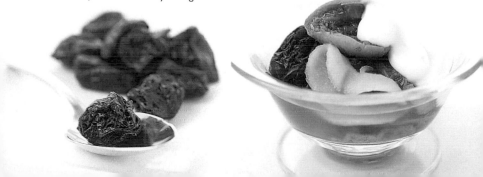

FOOD	CARB	FIBRE	FAT	ENERGY	
	g	g	g	kcal	kJ
GUAVA					
canned in juice, 100g	15.7	3	0	60	258
raw, 1 medium, 100g	5	3.7	0.5	26	112
HAGGIS boiled, 100g	19.2	N	21.7	310	1292
HALVA 30g	14.5	+	5	102	430
HAM					
& chicken luncheon meat, 2 slices, 23g	1	N	4	53	225
leg, canned, 2 slices, 35g	0	0	1.5	39	165
leg, fresh, lean, 2 slices, 46g	0	0	1.5	50	210
leg, fresh, untrimmed, 2. slices, 50g	0	0	4	70	295
light, 90% fat-free, 2 slices, 50g	0	0	2.5	36	150
shoulder, 2 slices, 50g	0	0	3	55	230
shoulder, canned, 2 slices, 35g	0	0	2	42	175
steak, grilled, 1, 115g	0	0	9	186	780
HAMBURGER (see FAST FOOD)					
HERBS					
average all varieties, dried, 1tbsp	Tr	N	0	19	80
average all varieties, fresh, chopped, 1tbsp	Tr	N	0	17	70
HONEY 1tbsp	22	0	0	84	355
HONEYCOMB 1 piece, 30g	22.2	0	1.5	86	360
HORSERADISH					
cream, 1tbsp	2.5	0.2	2	32	135
fresh, 5g	0.5	0.3	0.5	8	35
HUMMUS average serving, 100g	11.6	2.4	12.6	187	781
ICE CREAM BLOCK					
chocolate, 1, 158ml	36.5	0	0	150	630
neopolitan, 100ml	20	0	0	88	370
fruit-flavoured, 100ml	12.5	0	1	67	280
ICE CREAM					
caramel, 1	18	0	6	133	560
chocolate bar type, 1	21	0	19	260	1090
chocolate, 100ml	23	0	11.5	208	875
cone, large, vanilla, 1, 70g	24	0	12.5	220	925
cone, chocolate, 1, 70g	23	0	13.5	226	950
cone, single, plain wafer type, 1, 15g	4	0	0	19	80
cone, sugar, 1, 10g	8.5	0	0.5	40	170
cone, waffle, 1, 18g	3.5	0	0	15	65
cone with 1 small scoop ice cream	8.5	0	3	64	270
cone with 1 small scoop reduced-fat ice cream	8.5	0	1.5	54	225
fruits of the forest, 1, 86ml	20	0	6	142	595
lemon, 86ml	18.5	0	6	137	575
mango, 100ml	21	0	8	168	705
raspberry, 1, 90ml	17.5	0	3.5	107	450
soft-serve, 1, 100ml	21.5	0	4.5	137	575
stick, chocolate flavoured, 1, 90ml	19	0	3.5	126	530
stick, vanilla, chocolate coated, 1, 93ml	20.5	0	17.5	248	1040
stick, Belgian chocolate coated ice cream 1, 120ml	43	0	27	432	1815
tub, fruit cream, 100ml	10	+	5	94	395

HERBS

Adding herbs to your food is a healthy way to enhance the flavour of dishes without loading on the fat and salt. Many people also claim that herbs have medicinal properties and many of today's medical drugs do indeed come from plants. If you are interested in herbal medicine, try some herbal teas, which are now widely available.

BASIL Delicious with tomato dishes and the essential ingredient in pesto, basil is said to have a calming effect and aid digestion. Try basil tea after a rich meal or to relieve nausea.

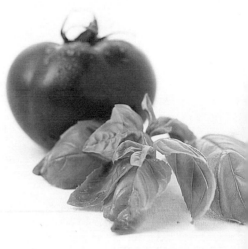

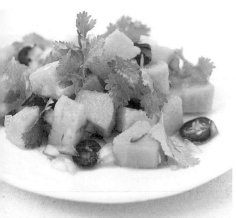

RECIPE Make a healthy fresh salsa from some ginger, pawpaw, chilli, red onion and coriander leaves. Serve with chicken or fish.

PARSLEY High in vitamins A and C, it is delicious with egg and seafood dishes. Also a great sugarless breath freshener.

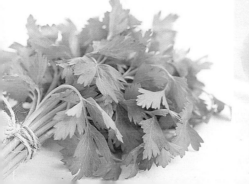

ROSEMARY May help to relieve indigestion. To add a subtle rosemary flavour to grilled meat, tie some rosemary sprigs together and use for basting.

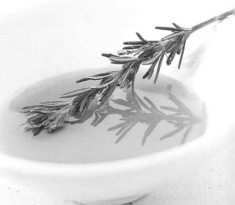

FOOD	CARB	FIBRE	FAT	ENERGY	
	g	g	g	kcal	kJ
ICE CREAM CONT.					
tub, chocolate, 100ml	9.5	0	5.5	92	385
tub, cookies & fudge,100ml	14.5	0	16	215	905
tub, light & creamy vanilla, 100ml	15	0	1.5	77	325
tub, natural vanilla, 100ml	10	0	6	101	425
tub, original vanilla, 100ml	10	0	4.8	89	375
tub, original extra creamy vanilla, 100ml	10.5	0	5.5	99	415
tub, strawberries & cream, 100ml	22.5	0	10.5	198	830
tub, double choc, 100ml	21	0	13.5	218	915
tub, vanilla choc-chip, 100ml	N	0	6	106	445
tub, vanilla light, 100ml	12	0	3	83	350
vanilla, 100ml	21	0	10	187	785
viennetta style, chocolate, 100ml	13	0	9	133	559
viennetta style, toffee, 100ml	13	0	10	129	540
viennetta style, vanilla, 100ml	13	0	10	124	520
JAM					
apricot, reduced sugar, 1tbsp	4	+	0	17	70
average, all types, 1tbsp	17	+	0	67	280
berry, 1tbsp	17.5	+	0	68	285
fruits of the forest, reduced sugar, 1tbsp	4	+	0	17	70
marmalade, orange, 1tbsp	17	+	0	65	275
marmalade, reduced sugar, 1tbsp	4	+	0	17	70
JELLY					
jelly, low-sugar, prepared, 1 bowl, 270ml	0	0	0	24	100
jelly, prepared, 1 bowl, 280ml	45.5	0	0	188	790
JUICE (see INDIVIDUAL FRUITS)					
KALE					
cooked, 65g	3.5	1.5	0.5	18	75
raw, 35g	3.5	1	0	18	75
KIWI FRUIT raw, peeled, 1 small, 75g	7.5	1.5	0	36	150
KOHL RABI peeled, boiled, 50g	2.5	1	0	18	75
LAMB					
chump chop, lean, grilled, 1, 55g	0	0	4.5	111	465
chump chop, untrimmed, grilled, 1, 65g	0	0	12	182	765
cutlet lean, grilled or baked, 1, 30g	0	0	4	70	295
cutlet, untrimmed, grilled or baked, 1, 40g	0	0	10.5	131	550
heart, baked, 70g	0	0	5.5	129	540
kidney, simmered, 150g	0	0	6.5	218	915
leg, lean, baked, 2 slices, 80g	0	0	5	158	665
leg, untrimmed, baked, 2 slices, 90g	0	0	10.5	201	845
liver, fried, 40g	0	0	5.5	96	405
loin chop, lean, grilled, 1, 35g	0	0	2.5	62	260
loin chop, untrimmed, grilled, 1, 50g	0	0	15.5	182	765
neck chop, lean, stewed, 1, 40g	0	0	5.5	101	425
neck chop, untrimmed, stewed, 1, 50g	0	0	14	176	740
shank, lean, cooked, 1, 130g	0	0	4.5	180	755
shank, untrimmed, cooked, 1, 100g	0	0	10.5	223	935
shoulder, lean, baked, 1 slice, 25g	0	0	2	46	195

LOW-FAT FROZEN FRUIT DESSERTS Sometimes with less than 2g fat per serving, these desserts are guilt-free and come in a variety of flavours.

SORBET With no fat, this is a refreshing, but sweet, alternative to ice cream. Usually made with fruit, so it can be high in vitamin C.

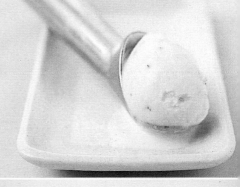

ICE CREAM As a general rule, the creamier the ice cream is, the higher the fat content. Ice cream is a good source of vitamins and calcium, but the milk or cream does add saturated fat. There are now many alternatives to ice cream in our supermarkets, including frozen fruit, tofu or yoghurt desserts – look out for the low-fat varieties.

GOURMET ICE CREAMS These often contain more fat than ordinary ice creams, but they are made with better-quality ingredients and sometimes contain real fruit.

RECIPE For a tasty and quick dessert, layer a passionfruit, fat-free frozen dessert with sliced banana and a spoonful of low-fat honey vanilla yoghurt. Top with some chopped nuts.

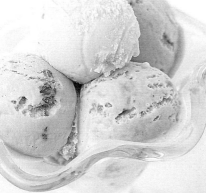

FOOD	CARB	FIBRE	FAT	ENERGY	
	g	g	g	kcal	kJ
LAMB CONT.					
shoulder, untrimmed, baked, 1 slice, 30g	0	0	6	87	365
trim, butterfly steak, grilled, 100g	0	0	4.5	125	525
trim, fillet, grilled, 100g	0	0	4	115	485.
trim, roast loin, baked, 100g	0	0	4	119	500
trim, schnitzel steak, grilled, 100g	0	0	3.5	111	465
strips, grilled, 100g	0	0	3.5	114	480
LASAGNE (see also PASTA)					
beef, commercial, 400g	62.8	2.8	24	572	2412
bolognaise, 400g	67.5	+	11.5	481	2020
lean beef lasagne, 400g	64	+	8.5	440	1850
LEEK sliced, boiled, 1 serving, 45g	1.2	0.8	0.3	9	39
LEMON					
curd, 1tbsp	10.5	0	3.5	76	320
juice, 100 ml	2.5	0	0	26	110
flavoured-spread, 1tbsp	13	0	1	60	250
raw, whole, 1, 65g	2.1	+	0	12	51
LENTILS					
burger, 1, 70g	15.5	2	1.5	213	895
dhal, 125g	14	2.5	9	177	745
dried, boiled, 200g	35	3.8	0.8	200	848
LETTUCE					
cos, 1 serving, 35g	0.6	0.3	0	6	25
iceberg, 35g	0.6	0.3	0	2	10
average, 35g	0.6	0.3	0	5	21
LIME					
juice, 1tbsp	2	0	0	6	25
raw, peeled, whole, 1, 45g	0.5	+	0	9	40
LINSEEDS (FLAXSEEDS) 1tbsp	4	+	4	58	245
LIQUORICE					
allsorts, 6, 56g	43	1	1.2	195	821
pieces, 5, 65g	42	1	1	181	759
LIVERWURST 60g	0.5	+	17.5	198	830
LOGANBERRIES raw, 100g	13	2.4	0.5	55	230
LOQUATS 6 medium, 78g	4	+	0	20	85
LOTUS ROOT					
canned, cooked, 100g	16	+	0	65	275
raw, peeled, 100g	17	+	0	74	310
LYCHEES					
canned in syrup, drained, 100g	17.7	0.5	0	68	290
raw, peeled, 100g	14.3	0.7	0.1	58	248
MACARONI					
cheese, homemade, 1 serving, 150g	20.4	0.8	16.2	267	1115
cheese, bought, 1 serving, 243g	49	1	15.5	405	1700
cheese, traditional, canned, 1 serving, 335g	71	1	21	557	2340
cheese & bacon, 1 serving, 293g	58	1	21	476	2000
cheesy fun shapes, 1 serving, 335g	71	1	21	557	2340
plain, boiled, 1 serving, 100g	18.5	0.9	0.5	86	365

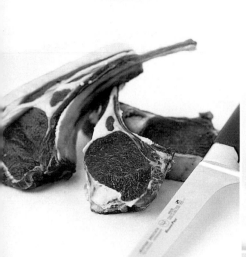

TRIM LAMB For a very lean cut of lamb, try eye of loin or backstrap. Avoid overcooking as lean cuts tend to dry out. Add to a stir-fry or try searing under the grill.

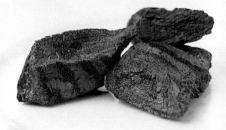

CUTTING FAT OFF LAMB When buying lamb, check how much fat you can see and whether it can be removed – a lamb cutlet that has been trimmed will have a lot less saturated fat. The leanest cuts are the leg and shank, the fattiest are the shoulder and rack.

DICED LAMB To make sure your diced lamb is lean, purchase lean cuts such as fillet or eye of loin and dice your own.

LAMB Although lamb was once considered to be a very fatty meat, changes in farming and breeding techniques have produced much leaner lamb that is widely available. Average, well-trimmed lamb can contain less than 8% fat, which is no more than many cuts of beef or pork. It's also worth trying out healthier methods of cooking, such as grilling, rather than just roasting.

RECIPE For no-fuss, low-fat lamb, marinate trimmed lamb cutlets in tandoori paste, lemon juice and plain low-fat yoghurt overnight. Grill until tender.

FOOD	CARB	FIBRE	FAT	ENERGY	
	g	g	g	kcal	kJ
MANDARIN					
canned in juice, drained, 1 serving, 100g	7.7	0.3	0	32	135
peeled, whole, 1, 60g	5	1	0	24	100
MANGO					
canned in syrup, 200g	40.6	1.4	0	144	660
chutney, 1tbsp	8.5	0.5	0	34	145
green, 150g	25	3	0	58	245
ripe, raw, peeled, whole, 1, 150g	21.2	3.9	0.3	86	368
MARGARINE					
average, 1 portion, 11g	0.1	0	9	81	334
light, salt-reduced, 11g	0	0	4	36	150
lite, 1tsp, 5g	0	0	3	26	110
sunflower spread, 11g	0.1	0	7.3	67	274
dairy blend, extra-soft, 1tsp, 5g	0	0	3	26	110
blended, 1tsp, 5g	0	0	3.5	31	130
butter type, 1tsp, 5g	0	0	4	36	150
high polyunsaturated spread, 1tsp	0	0	4	33	140
olive oil, type, 1tsp, 5g	0	0	4	33	140
sunflower spread, fat-reduced,					
1 tsp, 5g	0	0	2.5	21	90
MARROW					
peeled, boiled, 100g	4	0.5	0	19	80
raw, peeled, 100g	3.5	0.5	0	17	70
MARZIPAN 20g	11	0.6	3.5	80	335
MATZO					
meal, 50g	40	+	0	171	720
plain cracker, 30g	25	1	0.5	118	495
MAYONNAISE					
97% fat free, 1tbsp	9	0	20	45	190
cholesterol free, 1tbsp	7.5	0	3.5	63	265
sunflower type, 1tbsp	7.5	0	7.5	107	450
light, 1tbsp	8	0	7	63	265
olive oil type, 1tbsp	5	0	8.5	97	410
premium type, 1tbsp	7	0	3	58	245
traditional, 1tbsp	3	0	21.5	201	845
reduced calorie, 1tbsp	7	0	3	55	230
MEAT SUBSTITUTES					
micro protein, 100g	2	4.8	3.5	86	360
vegetarian mince, 100g	22	1.4	2.5	304	1280
MELON					
casaba, raw, peeled, 100g	6	0.4	0	32	135
honeydew, raw, peeled, 160g	10.5	0.6	0.5	50	210
rock, raw, peeled, 250g	12	1	0	55	230
water, raw, peeled, 100g	5	0.2	0	23	95
MERINGUE 25g	22.5	0	0	92	385
MILK					
buttermilk, cultured, dairy, 1 carton, 250ml	4	0	5.5	132	555
calcium enriched, 1 cup, 250ml	12.5	0	2.5	119	500

MILK Even whole cows' milk, which contains about 4% fat, would be classified as 'low fat' according to government guidelines. It is an excellent source of calcium and protein and also contains vitamins and minerals. Milk is an essential part of many people's diet, and is particularly important for infants and young children.

WHOLE MILK Relatively high in saturated fat, whole milk does contain more vitamin A and D than skimmed varieties.

CALCIUM It is recommended that adults consume 700mg calcium every day, in order to maintain healthy bones. This is about the amount available in a pint of milk (any variety).

RECIPE For a lactose-free alternative to milk, place almonds or cashews in a blender and process until fine. Add boiling or cold water and a pitted date and blend until smooth. Sprinkle with nutmeg.

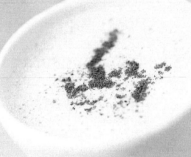

SKIMMED MILK Although this lacks the fat-soluble vitamins A and D, skimmed milk has the same amount of calcium as other varieties.

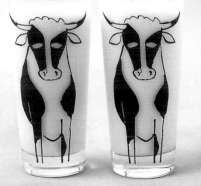

SEMI-SKIMMED MILK With 50–60% less fat than whole milk, this is an excellent means of cutting down on fat and still maintaining calcium levels.

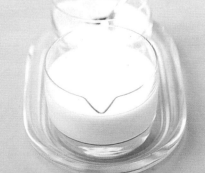

FOOD	CARB	FIBRE	FAT	ENERGY	
	g	g	g	kcal	kJ
MILK CONT.					
condensed, sweetened, 1 tin, 250ml	180	0	30	1060	4455
condensed, sweetened, skim, 250ml	199	0	1	901	3785
cultured, reduced-fat, 250ml	12	0	5	134	565
cultured, skim, 250ml	14.5	0	0.5	108	455
evaporated, reduced-fat, canned, 250ml	28.5	0	5.5	241	1015
evaporated, skim, canned, 250ml	28.5	0	1	200	840
evaporated, whole-fat, canned, 250ml	27	0	21.5	373	1565
fat-reduced, protein-increased, 250ml	14	0	3.5	126	530
flavoured, chocolate, 250ml	23	0	9.5	204	855
flavoured, chocolate, reduced-fat, 1 cup, 250ml	21.5	0	4.5	156	655
flavoured, malt & honey, 250ml	27	0	2.5	170	715
flavoured, strawberry, 250ml	23	0	9	201	845
flavoured, strawberry, reduced-fat, 250ml	24	0	4	158	665
full-cream, 250ml	12	0	10	167	700
goat's, 1 cup, 250ml	9.5	0	6.5	127	535
lite, 250ml	14.5	0	3.5	133	558
low-fat, high-calcium, 250ml	17	0	0.5	120	505
milkshake, 275ml	47	0	12	349	1465
milkshake, thick, 300ml	60	0	10	355	1490
powder, malted, 1tbsp	5.5	0	0.5	32	135
powdered, full-cream, 1tbsp	3	0	2	39	165
powdered, skim, 1tbsp	4	0	0	29	120
rice, 250ml	N	0	2.5	157	660
sheep's, 250ml	13.5	0	17.5	268	1125
skimmed, 250ml	12.5	0	0.5	88	370
soya, natural, 250ml	18.5	+	7	158	665
soya, low-fat, 250ml	12	N	1.8	91	382
soya, lite, 250ml	15	N	1.5	107	450
soya, flavoured, banana, 250ml	23	+	2	138	580
soya, flavoured, chocolate hazelnut, 250ml	18.5	5	7	158	665
MILLET					
cooked, 174g	41	+	1.5	206	865
MISO (SOYA BEAN PASTE) 1tbsp	6	+	1	40	170
MIXED PEEL 100g	59	4.8	1	231	984
MIXED VEGETABLES					
frozen, boiled, 1 serving 100g	6.6	+	0.5	42	180
MOLASSES 1tbsp	14	0	0	54	225
MUESLI (see CEREAL)					
MUESLI BAR (see also CEREAL BAR)					
apricot & coconut, 1 bar, 31g	19.5	N	7.5	149	625
apricot & fibre, yoghurt-coated bar,					
1 bar, 50g	28	+	9.5	202	850
brown rice, macadamia & ginger, 1 bar, 50g	26	+	14	234	985
chewy fruit, 1 bar, 31g	21	1	5	131	550
crunchy fruit, 1 bar, 31g	17.5	1.2	7	146	615
crunchy original, yoghurt, 1 bar, 31g	22	+	4	126	530
fruit, apricot, 1 bar, 32g	22.5	+	4.5	137	575

BUTTERMILK A low-fat alternative to milk, buttermilk has a slightly sour taste and can be used in cooking to replace whole milk.

SOYA MILK As it is not a natural source of calcium, many varieties have calcium added. However, they may also be sweetened so avoid frequent consumption.

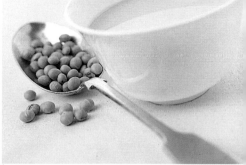

EVAPORATED MILK This is milk that has had much of its water evaporated. Look for low-fat varieties, which can replace cream in cooking.

MILK Although dairy products are an important part of a healthy diet, they are also relatively high in saturated fat and should be consumed in moderation. However, simply cutting back on dairy products may result in a lower calcium intake, so instead try replacing them with lower fat alternatives, which will not affect calcium levels.

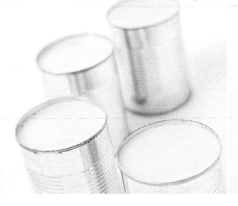

RICE MILK A high-carbohydrate drink, rice milk is a good option for those who are lactose-intolerant. It is sweeter than soy milk.

MILK POWDER This loses little of the nutritional value associated with normal milk.

FOOD	CARB	FIBRE	FAT	ENERGY	
	g	g	g	kcal	kJ
MUESLI BAR CONT.					
nut crumble, 1 bar, 31g	20	+	6	143	600
nut & muesli, carob-coated, 1 bar, 50g	28	+	11	218	915
peach & pear, 100% fruit, 1 bar, 25g	15	N	8.6	131	550
yoghurt, apricot, 1 bar, 31g	20.5	+	5.5	138	580
yoghurt tops, fruit salad, 1 bar, 31g	21.5	+	5	136	570
MUFFIN					
1 medium, plain, 60g	29	1.5	8	169	710
1 large, 100g	48	2	13	279	1170
1 extra large, 150g	72	3	19.5	418	1755
blueberry, 1 , 150g	56	+	13	352	1480
bran, 1, 190g	67	15	27.5	550	2310
calorie-reduced, 1, 152g	47.5	+	18	370	1555
high-fibre, 1, 63g	27.5	+	2	152	640
fruit, 1, 60g	27	+	1.5	151	635
soya & linseed, 1, 67g	N	++	6.5	180	755
spicy fruit topped, 1, 67g	30	+	2	168	705
white, bread type, 1, 67g	28.5	2	1	151	635
wholemeal, bread type, 1, 67g	N	+	2	156	655
low-fat, 1, 152g	57.5	+	2.5	283	1190
mixed berry, 1, 60g	38	+	5	207	870
muffin mix, apple & sultana, prepared, 1, 60g	33	+	7	202	850
muffin mix, blueberry & apricot, prepared, 1, 60g	32	+	6.7	202	850
muffin mix, choc-chip, prepared, 1, 60g	32	N	7	213	895
MULBERRIES					
raw, 100g	4.5	++	0	29	120
MUSHROOMS					
button, raw, 100g	1.5	1.1	0.5	24	100
canned, 100g	1.5	1.3	0.5	15	65
canned in butter sauce, 100g	3.5	1	1	27	115
champignon, canned, 100g	1	1	0	13	55
chinese, dried & rehydrated, 25g	4	N	0	14	60
enoki, raw, 100g	7	N	0.5	35	145
oyster, raw, 100g	6	+	0.5	37	155
shiitake, dried, 4, 15g	11	+	0	44	185
straw, canned, drained, 100g	4.5	+	0.5	32	135
swiss brown, 100g	N	+	0	23	95
MUSTARD					
American, 1tbsp	1	0	0	15	65
English, 1tbsp	1	0	0	15	65
French, 1tbsp	1	0	0	15	65
powder, wholegrain, 1tsp, 5g	0.5	1	1	18	75
seeded, 1tbsp	1	+	0	15	65
NASHI PEAR					
raw, unpeeled, 1, 130g	9.2	2	0	38	158
NECTARINE					
raw, unpeeled, 1, 75g	6.75	1	0	30	126

CAROB-COATED BARS An alternative to chocolate, carob has the same amount of fat but is free of caffeine.

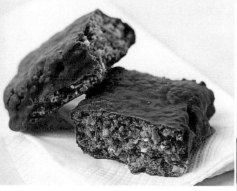

BREAKFAST BARS A good breakfast is a great way to start the day but if you don't have time, bars can be a convenient alternative to cereal.

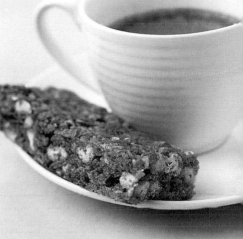

MUESLI & CEREAL BARS Often

eaten as a quick snack, muesli bars can be a good source of dietary fibre and may be a healthier snack option than a packet of crisps or a chocolate bar. However, they are not always as healthy as they seem and can contain up to 17g of fat and lots of sugar per bar. Check the label carefully.

MUESLI BARS Some varieties are high in sugar and provide a great energy boost when eaten before or after exercise. If you are not that active, they may provide more energy than you need.

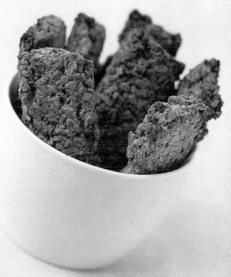

YOGHURT-COATED BARS Handy for a picnic or lunch box, some contain real fruit. Check the fat content on the label.

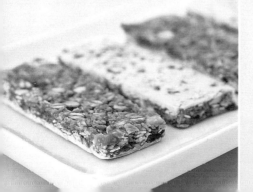

FOOD	CARB	FIBRE	FAT	ENERGY	
	g	g	g	kcal	kJ
NOODLES					
egg, boiled, 1 portion, 100g	13	0.6	0.5	62	264
instant, boiled, 1 portion, 100g	N	+	5	367	1540
rice, boiled, 1 portion, 100g	21.5	0.5	0.5	99	415
rice, fried, 1 portion, 150g	16.8	0.8	17.2	230	964
rice, vermicelli, boiled, 30g	N	+	0.5	110	460
buckwheat, boiled, 100g	21.5	+	0	99	415
quick-cook noodles, all flavours, 1 packet, 85g	54	+	16	390	1640
noodles, rice, dry, 100g	81.5	+	0.1	360	1506
wheat, fried, 80g	50	+	17	374	1570
wheat, steamed, 80g	60	+	2	283	1190
NUTMEAT					
canned, 100g	6	+	8.5	195	820
NUTS					
almond, blanched, 85g	5.8	6.3	47.5	520	2185
almond, chocolate-coated, 75g	49.5	4.5	33.5	517	2170
almond, raw, 4	0.5	1.5	8	87	365
almond, raw & unpeeled, 85g	2	2.3	17.5	195	817
almond, smoked, 30g	1.5	N	15	194	815
almond, sugar-coated, 30g	N	N	12	130	545
brazil, raw, 80g	2.5	3.4	54.5	546	2291
cashew, raw, 75g	13.6	2.4	36	430	1805
cashew, roasted, 75g	14	2.4	38	458	1925
chestnut, raw, 72g	26	3	2	122	514
hazelnut, raw, 70g	4.2	4.5	44.4	455	1911
macadamia, salted, 73g	3.5	3.8	56.6	546	2293
mixed, 78g	6	4.7	42	473	1988
mixed nuts & raisins, 100g	31.5	4.5	34	481	2004
peanut, raw, 78g	9.75	4.8	35.9	440	1848
peanut, roasted, 78g	8	5	38.8	459	1930
pecan, raw, 55g	3.2	2.6	38.5	379	1592
pinenut, raw, 1tbsp, 15g	0.6	0.3	10.2	103	433
pistachio, raw, 63g	5	3.8	35	379	1590
walnut chopped, raw, 55g	1.8	2	38	378	1589
OATMEAL 40g	29	2.7	3.5	160	674
OIL					
blended, 1tbsp	0	0	20	176	740
cod liver, 1tbsp	0	0	20	176	740
olive oil, 1tbsp	0	0	19	167	703
OKRA					
boiled, 6 pods, 65g	1	2.3	0	13	55
OLIVES					
black, 6 medium, 40g	N	N	7	39	165
green, 6 medium, 50g	Tr	1.5	5.5	56	211
stuffed, 5 olives, 20g	0.5	1.5	1.5	18	75
ONION					
brown, raw, peeled, 1 medium, 100g	4.5	1.4	0	24	100
pickled, drained, 2, 36g	4.5	0.4	0	21	90

RECIPE To make your own basil oil, simply heat some extra virgin olive oil, then add fresh herbs and cool. Process, then strain and use immediately.

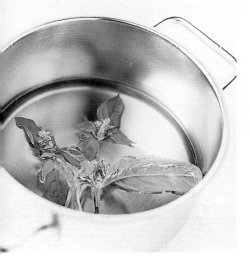

OIL All oils contain roughly the same amount of fat, but the important issue is the type of fat. Palm and coconut oils, often used for frying, are high in saturated fat and should be avoided, while the other oils have more monounsaturated and polyunsaturated fats, both of which have health benefits.

MONOUNSATURATED OILS These oils, such as olive, canola or peanut, are thought to lower blood cholesterol when they replace saturated fat in the diet.

POLYUNSATURATED OILS These oils, such as sunflower or corn oil, contain essential fatty acids that the body cannot produce itself. They may also lower blood cholesterol when they replace saturated fats in the diet.

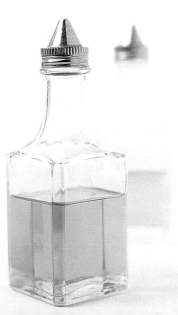

HOW MUCH? Oils contain 1g of fat to 1ml of oil, so they should be used in moderation. Oil sprays are a good way to make sure you use a small amount of oil.

FOOD	CARB	FIBRE	FAT	ENERGY	
	g	g	g	kcal	kJ
ONION CONT.					
red, raw, peeled, 1 small, 100g	4.5	1.4	0	25	105
spring, raw, whole, 1, 14g	0.5	0.2	0	3	14
white, raw, peeled, 1 medium, 100g	4.5	1.4	0	26	110
ORANGE					
all varieties, raw, peeled, 120g	10.2	2	0	44	186
juice, freshly squeezed, 100ml	8.1	0.1	0	33	140
juice, commercial, unsweetened, 100ml	8.8	0.1	0	36	153
PANCAKE					
average, homemade, 1, 16 cm, 50g	14	0.5	1	75	315
PAPADUM					
fried, 3 small, 10g	3.9	N	1.7	37	155
grilled or microwaved, 3 small	N	N	0	17	70
PAPAYA (PAWPAW)					
raw, peeled, 100g	8.8	2.2	0	36	153
canned in juice,100g	17	0.7	0	65	275
PARSNIP raw, peeled, boiled, 100g	12.9	4.7	1.2	66	278
PASSIONFRUIT 1 average, 40g	2.5	1.5	0	19	80
PASTA (see also LASAGNE AND SPAGHETTI)					
egg, cooked, 1 serving, 200g	51	2	1	261	1095.
plain, all shapes, cooked, 1 serving, 180g	44.5	1.8	0.5	213	895
ravioli, cheese & spinach, cooked, 1 serving, 265g	88	+	16.5	640	2690
ravioli, meat, cooked, 1 serving, 265g	82.5	+	17.5	602	2530
spinach, cooked, 1 serving, 200g	54.5	+	1	258	1085
tomato & herb fettucine, cooked, 200g	39	+	1.5	186	780
tortellini, cheese & spinach, cooked, 1 serving, 265g	88	+	16.5	640	2690
tortellini, meat, 1 serving	N	N	5	379	1590
wholemeal, cooked, 1 serving, 180g	42	6.3	1.6	203	854
PASTA SAUCE					
carbonara, jar, 1 serving, 125g	21.5	+	6.5	158	665
creamy mushroom, 1 serving, 280g	25	+	0.5	119	500
spicy tomato, 1 serving, 125g	20.5	+	5	140	589
tomato, bottled, 1 serving, 280g	26.5	+	2	134	565
PASTRY					
choux, cooked, 30g	9	0.4	7	108	454
filo, 2 sheets	15	N	0.5	77	325
flaky, average portion, cooked, 50g	23	0.9	20.3	280	1176
hot-water, 50g	27	N	10	213	895
puff, 1 sheet, 170g	63	N	42.3	671	2820
shortcrust, cooked, 100g	54.2	2.2	32.3	521	2174
strudel, 50g	23	N	20	267	1120
suet crust, 50g	27	N	10	213	895
wholemeal, cooked, 100g	44.6	6.3	32.9	499	2080
PATE					
chicken liver, 1tbsp	N	0	2.5	27	112
country, 1tbsp	0.5	0.5	5	59	250
PAVLOVA					
pavlova shell mix, prepared, 1 serving, 60g	4	0	0	173	725

RECIPE For a quick and healthy pasta sauce, cook a chopped onion and garlic clove in a non-stick pan until soft. Add a little red or white wine and some fresh chopped tomatoes and toss together until heated through. Sprinkle with slivers of Parmesan.

CREAMY SAUCES You can make low-fat versions of cream sauces like Alfredo and Carbonara using stock, low-fat milk and some cornflour to thicken.

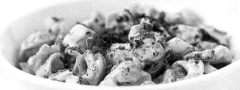

PASTA & PASTA SAUCE

High in starchy carbohydrates and low in fat, pasta is a healthy way to fill up. However, it's the pasta sauce that can pile on the fat and calories. Always serve plenty of pasta with only a relatively small amount of topping, and opt for a homemade tomato sauce, rather than high-fat creamy or cheesy sauces.

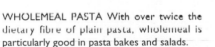

WHOLEMEAL PASTA With over twice the dietary fibre of plain pasta, wholemeal is particularly good in pasta bakes and salads.

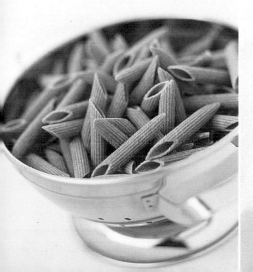

PLAIN PASTA Though the flour used to make plain pasta has had the wheatgerm and bran removed, it still contains plenty of fibre and starch.

FOOD	CARB	FIBRE	FAT	ENERGY	
	g	g	g	kcal	kJ
PAVLOVA CONT.					
shell, with cream & passion fruit, I serving	N	+	11	315	1325
PAWPAW whole, raw, 100g	7	2	0	30	125
PEACH					
canned in jelly, snack pack	N	N	0	95	400
canned in juice, drained, 140g	12.5	1.2	0	56	235
canned in syrup, 250g	14	2.2	0	61	255
dried, 25g	13	1.8	0	61	255
raw, I medium, 140g	9	2	0	44	185
stewed, with sugar, 100g	25.5	2.9	0.5	106	445
stewed, without sugar, 100g	21.5	3	0.5	92	385
PEAR					
canned, snack pack 140g	N	2	0	82	345
canned in pear juice, drained, 250g	25.5	3.5	0	106	445
canned in syrup, drained, 250g	37	2.75	0	148	620
canned in water, drained, 250g	16	3.5	0	64	270
dried, 2, 87g	60.5	7.2	0.5	227	955
juice, canned, 200ml	27.5	0	0	112	470
raw, unpeeled, 185g	18.5	4	0	74	311
PEAS					
green, cooked, I serving, 165g	10.5	7.4	0.5	80	335
peas, raw, 170g	10	8	1	98	410
split, dried, cooked, I serving, 180g	12	4.9	1	104	435
sugar snap, 170g	10	2.2	1	98	410
PHEASANT raw, meat only, 125g	0	0	4.5	165	695
PIGEON breast, lean, roasted, 125g	0	0	14.5	263	1105
PINEAPPLE					
canned in juice, drained, I bowl, 250ml	25.5	1.25	0	112	470
canned in syrup, drained, I slice, 40g	8	0.3	0	33	140
juice, unsweetened, canned, 250ml	27	0	0	111	465
raw, peeled, I slice, 110g	9	1.3	0	42	175
PIE meat, average,					
all types, 1, 190g	34	0.8	26	429	1800
PIZZA (see FAST FOOD)					
PLUM					
canned in syrup, drained, I serving, 225g	35	1.8	0.3	132	557
raw, 100g	8.8	1.6	0	36	155
stewed, without sugar, I serving, 250g	17	4	0	85	357
POLENTA dry, 60g	41	+	1	198	830.
POMEGRANATE raw, peeled, 100g	11.8	3.4	0.2	51	218
POPCORN					
caramel-coated, 100g	77.6	N	20	480	2018
plain, commercial, 2 scoops, 16g	8.5	N	4	75	315
PORK					
bacon, breakfast rasher, grilled, 1, 34g	0	0	1.5	48	200
barbecued, Chinese-style, 100g	3.5	N	15	233	980
belly, rasher, untrimmed, grilled, 100g	0	0	22	298	1250
crackling, 30g	0	0	9	142	610

PORK Thought of as a fatty meat, pork is now bred to be leaner. In fact, lean cuts of pork often have less fat than beef, lamb and chicken. However, other pork products, such as salami, sausages, spare ribs and bacon, have a much higher fat content in general, and are also quite high in saturated fat.

BACON The fat content of bacon can be reduced by up to 50%, simply by trimming off all visible fat and grilling rather than frying.

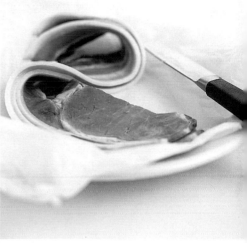

RECIPE To cook lean pork, fry lean steaks in a non-stick pan until brown and tender. Remove, then add some sliced apple, wholegrain mustard and apple cider to the pan. Simmer until the apples are soft, add the steaks and reheat.

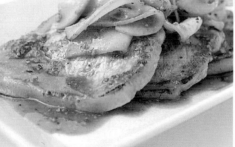

FILLET The leanest cut of pork, this is an excellent substitute for beef or lamb in stir-fries. Alternatively, cut the fillet into slices and grill or barbecue.

LEAN STEAKS Lean pork steaks are ideal for grilling or pan-frying with little or no added fat. Always remove visible fat before cooking.

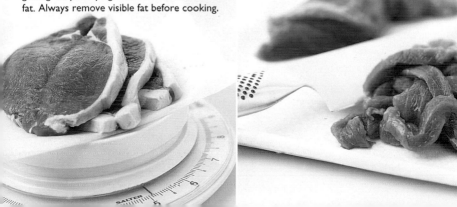

FOOD	CARB	FIBRE	FAT	ENERGY	
	g	g	g	kcal	kJ
PORK CONT.					
fillet lean, baked, 1, 100g	0	0	5	169	710
forequarter chop, lean, grilled, 1, 95g	0	0	7.5	171	720
forequarter chop, untrimmed, grilled, 1, 100g	0	0	28.5	343	1440
leg roast, lean, 2 slices, 95g	0	0	4	163	685
leg roast with fat, 2 slices, 100g	0	0	26.5	338	1420
leg, lean, grilled, 1, 100g	0	0	3.5	156	655
leg, untrimmed, grilled, 1, 100g	0	0	6	171	720
loin chop, lean, grilled. 1, 100g	0	0	5.5	174	730
loin chop, untrimmed, grilled, 1, 100g	0	0	30	362	1520
medallion steak, lean, grilled, 1 small, 100g	0	0	5.5	187	785
medallion steak, untrimmed, grilled,					
1 small, 100g	0	0	22.5	307	1290
mince, 100g	0	0	30	75	315
pie, 1, 180g	46.5	1.8	53.5	763	3205
ribs, spare, 100g	0	0	10	114	480
steak, lean, grilled, 100g	0	0	4.5	161	675
steak untrimmed, grilled, 100g	0	0	17.5	259	1090
POTATO					
baked, jacket, no oil, 1 medium, 150g	21.5	2	1	109	460
boiled, peeled, 1 medium, 150g	19.5	1.5	0.5	96	405
boiled, unpeeled, 1 medium, 150g	20	2	0	98	410
chips, oven-cook, frozen, cooked, 100g	25	2	3	131	550
fries (thin-cut), medium serving	43	1	18	338	1420
oven-fried, 100g	29	6	13	245	1030
hash brown, 1 average, 55g	15	1	12	171	720
mashed with milk & butter, 1 serving, 120g	N	2.5	1	77	325
mashed with skim milk, 120g	N	2.5	0	71	300
new, peeled, boiled, 3, 165g	21	3	0	103	435
roast, no skin, 150g	26	2.5	4	159	670
roast, with skin. 150g	25	2	4	159	670
steamed, new, peeled, 165g	20	3	0	102	430
wedges, crunchy, 100g	26	4.5	6	165	695
POTATO CRISPS					
(see CORN CHIPS AND SNACK FOOD)					
PRICKLY PEAR raw, peeled, 86g	7.5	N	0	34	145
PRUNES					
dried, 5, 38g	16.5	2.2	0	70	295
juice, 250ml	44.5	Tr	0	181	760.
stewed, with sugar, 150g	29.5	4.6	0	119	500
stewed, without sugar, 150g	18.5	4.8	0	78	330
PUMPKIN					
peeled, boiled, 85g	6	1	0.5	36	150
pie, 1 slice, 109g	29.5	3	10.5	229	960
roasted in oil with ½tbsp oil, 85g	8	1.5	8	125	525
seeds, dry roasted, 1tbsp	4.5	1	11.5	134	565
PURSLANE					
boiled, 1 cup, 115g	4	N	0	20	85

WEDGES For a healthy alternative to chips, lightly spray potato wedges with oil and bake in a 200°C (400°F/Gas 6) oven for 40 minutes until golden.

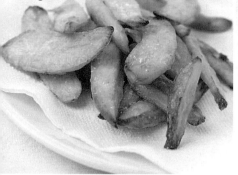

POTATO High in carbohydrate, potassium and vitamin C, potatoes are a great staple food – it's just the way they're cooked, and their affinity with butter and salt, that can make them unhealthy. Baking is a healthy way to cook potatoes. Boiled potatoes are also low in fat, but some of the vitamin C may be lost in the cooking water.

MASH You can make delicious mashed potatoes without too much butter. Use skimmed milk or stock, or try adding a little olive oil instead of the butter.

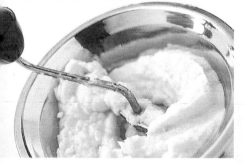

STEAMING A great way to cook potatoes and retain more vitamin C than boiling. Add some fresh herbs rather than lots of butter and salt.

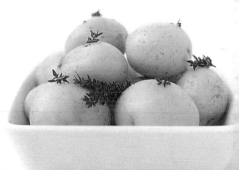

NEW POTATOES There are many potato varieties now available. Make a delicious salad with new potatoes and fresh herbs.

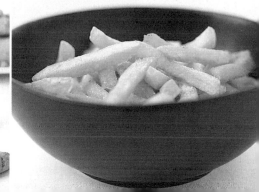

FRIES Fried potatoes are all fatty, but the thicker the chip, the less fat is absorbed during cooking. If you love fries, choose wedges.

FOOD	CARB	FIBRE	FAT	ENERGY	
	g	g	g	kcal	kJ
QUAIL					
roasted, with skin, 180g	0	0	6	180	755
roasted, without skin, 125g	0	0	20	349	1465
QUICHE					
cheese & egg, average homemade,					
slice, 125g	21.5	1	27.5	390	1640
lorraine, average, 100g	18	N	22	293	1230
mushroom, average homemade, 1 slice, 125g	23	1.5	24.5	352	1480
vegetable, average, 100g	20	N	18	259	1090
QUINCE					
raw, 100g	11	++	0	48	200
stewed, with added sugar, 100g	21	+	0	83	350
RABBIT meat only, baked, 100g	0	0	5.5	169	710
RADISH					
red, raw, 3, 45g	1	0.5	0	0.6	2.5
white, raw, peeled, sliced, 90g	2.5	1.5	0.5	15	65
RAISINS 100g	69.3	2	0.4	272	1159
RASPBERRIES					
canned in syrup, drained, 100g	22.5	1.5	0	88	374
raw, 65g	3	1.6	0.2	16	71
REDCURRANTS raw, 100g	14	3.4	0	56	235
RELISH					
corn, 1tbsp	4.5	0.2	0	20	85
mustard, 1tbsp	4.5	N	0	20	85
tomato, 1tbsp	4.5	0.2	0	19	80
RHUBARB					
raw, 100g	0.8	1.4	0	7	32
stewed with sugar, 125g	14.5	1.5	0	60	252
RICE					
average, cooked, 100g	33.4	0.1	1.1	157	660
basmati, cooked, 1 serving	42	+	0.3	177	742
brown, cooked, 1 serving, 180g	57	1.5	2	270	1135
extra-long grain, cooked, 70g	54.5	0.5	0.5	232	973
fragrant, cooked, 100g	34.6	0.5	0.4	155	651
fried, 190g	56	1.1	16	413	1735
long grain, cooked, 100g	34.6	+	0.4	155	651
white, cooked, 1 serving, 190g	53	0.2	0.5	237	995
wild, cooked, 1 serving, 164g	35	+	N	165	695
RICE CAKES					
corn & buckwheat, 1, 12g	10	+	0	49	205
corn cakes, natural, 2, 10g	9	+	0	36	150
natural brown, 2, 10g	8	+	0.5	14	60
rice & rye, 2, 10g	8	+	0.5	39	165
SAFFRON 1tbsp	1.5	0	0	6	25
SALADS					
bean salad, commercial, 1 serving, 210g	27	6.3	18	309	1298
coleslaw, commercial, 1 carton, 200g	8.4	2.8	52.8	516	1872
potato salad, 1 carton, 180g	20.5	1.4	47	517	1913

RICE

The main staple of half the people in the world and an excellent source of energy, rice makes the perfect accompaniment to any meal as it gives a feeling of fullness without adding fat. When mixed with legumes, rice forms a complete protein, which is particularly important for vegetarians. It is also a gluten-free alternative to bread.

WHITE RICE The bran layer is removed during processing, leaving white rice lower in thiamin than wholegrain rice.

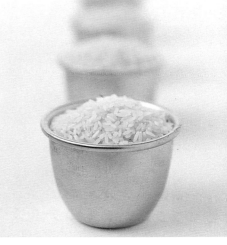

RECIPE Next time you make a soup, add some cooked rice to it. It will help to thicken it and raise carbohydrate levels.

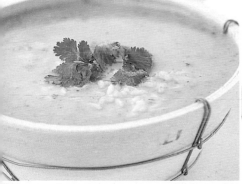

WILD RICE Not a true rice, but a grass native to North America. It can be blended with brown or white rice to add a delicious nutty flavour to dishes.

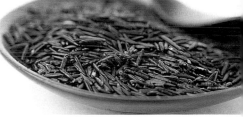

RICE PREFERENCES Although white varieties of rice may contain less fibre than wholegrain types, they are still nutritious and many people prefer the less distinctive flavour.

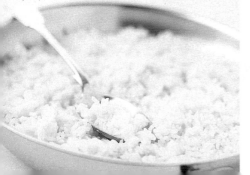

WHOLEGRAIN RICE This contains more fibre than white varieties. Although it can take longer to cook, it has a delicious, nutty flavour.

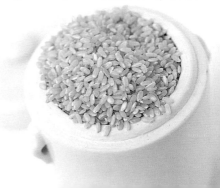

FOOD	CARB	FIBRE	FAT	ENERGY	
	g	g	g	kcal	kJ
SALAMI					
average, all varieties, 50g	0.5	0	19	214	900
Danish, 4 slices, 20g	0.5	N	8	88	370
pepperoni, 4 slices, 20g	0.5	0	7	80	335
SAUCES					
mayonnaise, 1tbsp	0.1	0	13	118	495
apricot chicken, 1 serving, 118g	15	0	1	69	290
apricot chicken, jar, 1 serving, 115g	16	0	10.5	67	280
barbecue, 1 tbsp	10	0	0	40	170
beef & black bean, 115g	11	0	1.5	58	245
bolognaise, 160g	3.5	N	14	192	805
butterscotch, 45g	15	0	17	214	900
chilli, 20g	10.5	0	0	9	40
country French chicken, 118g	5	0	11.5	126	530
creamy lemon chicken, 118g	15	0	0.7	69	290
creamy mushroom, 1 serving, 120g	6.5	0	1.5	133	560
golden honey mustard, 118g	12	0	13	170	715
gravy, commercial, 60g	5.5	0	5.5	81	340
gravy, made from powder, prepared, 60g	2.5	0	0	14	60
herbed chicken & wine, 1 serving, 115g	7.5	0	6.5	14	60
honey & sesame, 1 serving, 120g	23	0	1	108	455
honey, sesame & garlic, 1 serving, 115g	23	0	0.5	85	400
Hungarian goulash, 1 serving, 125g	7.5	0	3.5	105	440
Malaysian satay, 1tbsp	5	+	5	67	280
mild Indian, 1 serving, 115g	8	0	7	93	390
mint homemade, 1 tbsp	0	0	0	9	40
mornay, bought, 1 serving, 120g	5	0	14	161	675
onion, made from powdered mix, prepared, 125g	8.5	0	7	110	460
oyster, 1 tbsp	5	0	0	29	120
packet, average all types, 1 serving, 125g	10	0	20	263	1105
pesto, 1 tbsp	9	+	5	90	380
soya, 1 tbsp	0.5	0	0	9	40
spicy plum, 1 serving, 115g	21	N	0.5	86	360
sweet & sour, 1 serving, 115g	30.5	N	0	120	505
sweet & sour, lite, 1 serving, 115g	20.5	N	0	80	335
sweet Thai chilli, 115g	52.5	N	0.5	204	855
toffee, 1, 20g	15	0	2	80	335
tomato, 1tbsp	5.5	+	0	23	95
white, homemade, 1tbsp	2.5	+	5	27	115
worcestershire, 1tbsp	4	0	0	17	70
SAUSAGE					
beef, fried, homemade, 1, 50g	2	0.3	9	117	490
beef, grilled, homemade, 1, 50g	3	0.3	9	127	535
Bierschinken, 1, 30g	0	0	5	309	1300
black pudding, grilled, 1, 90g	6.5	+	21	281	1180
bratwurst, 100g	0	0	30	362	1520
cabanossi, 1, 30g	0	N	10	109	460
chicken, thin, 2, 50g	0	0	6	89	375

WHITE SAUCE For a low-fat alternative to this creamy sauce, use skimmed milk and replace the flour and butter with cornflour.

TOMATO SAUCE High in sugar and sodium, but lower in fat than mayonnaise-based sauces.

SAUCES If you are using a small

quantity of a sauce like tomato ketchup, you don't need to worry too much about its nutritional value. However, some sauces, especially cheesy or creamy sauces, can be high in fat. Ready-made commercial sauces tend also to be high in salt. Where possible, make your own, healthy varieties.

RECIPE Make your own tomato sauce by simmering some ripe tomatoes, vinegar and a little sugar. Use herbs for added flavour and store in sterilized jars.

COOK-IN SAUCES Can be high in fat and additives, so check the labels. Next time you make a tomato sauce, freeze half so you can add to meat or pasta for an instant dinner.

MINT SAUCE Make your own low-calorie version by mixing a handful of chopped mint leaves with a teaspoon of sugar, boiling water, and 3–4 tablespoons of white wine vinegar.

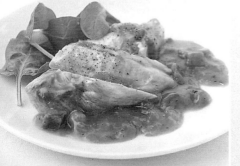

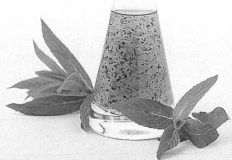

FOOD	CARB	FIBRE	FAT	ENERGY	
	g	g	g	kcal	kJ
SAUCES CONT.					
chicken, thin, low-fat, 2, 40g	0	0	3	70	295
chipolates (skinless), 2, 25g	0	0	5	55	230
Italian, cooked, 100g	0	0	30	362	1520
Chinese sausage, 100g	3	0	40	429	1800
low-fat, 1, 50g	0	0	5	75	315
pork, thick, grilled, 2, 150g	9	1	33	425	1785
pork, thin, grilled, 2, 100g	6	0.7	21.5	283	1190
Schinkenwurst, 30g	0	0	15	154	645
vegetarian, 1, 60g	4	1	4	98	410
SCONE					
fruit, 1, 50g	20	+	3	118	495
plain, average, 1, 50g	23	1	5	154	645
SEAFOOD					
baked, 85g	0	0	1	95	400
anchovies, canned in oil, drained, 5, 18g	0	0	1.5	33	140
bass, 100g	0	0	1	93	390
blackfish, 100g	0	0	2	93	390
blue grenadier, 100g	0	0	2	93	390
blue threadfin, 100g	0	0	2	93	390
boarfish, 100g	0	0	2	93	390
bream, steamed, 1 fillet, 149g	0	0	8	206	865
calamari tubes, raw, 100g	0	0	0	69	290
calamari tubes, fried, 100g	12	N	17.5	276	1160
caviar, black, 1tbsp, 16g	0.5	0	3	40	170
caviar, red, 1tbsp, 16g	0.5	0	3	40	170
clams, 100g	0	N	2	81	340
cockles, raw, 100g	0	0	0	48	200
cod, baked, 100g	0	0	1	76	320
cod, grilled, 100g	0	0	2	95	400
cod, poached, 100g	0	0	2	95	400
cod, smoked, simmered, 1 fillet, 195g	0	0	1.5	89	375
crab, all varieties, 90g	0	0	0.5	54	230
crab, canned in brine, 145g	2	0	1	88	370
eel, 85g	0	0	12.5	190	800
eel, smoked, 100g	10	0	13	167	700
fish ball, boiled, 1, 50g	2	0	0.5	37	155
fish paste, 1tbsp, 20g	2	0	1.5	31	130
fish roe, black, 1tbsp, 20g	0	0	1	18	75
fish roe, red, 1tbsp, 20g	0	0	1.5	30	125
fish, steamed, 1 small fillet, 85g	0	0	2.5	105	440
flake, crumbed & fried, 1 fillet, 165g	10.5	+	8.5	293	1230
flake, steamed, 1 fillet, 150g	0	0	0	187	785
flathead, fried, 1 fillet, 104g	3.5	0	7	183	770
flathead, steamed, 1 fillet, 85g	0	0	1	96	405
flounder, 100g	0	0	1	67	280
garfish, 100g	0	0	2	93	390
gemfish, 1 fillet, 175g	0	0	27	393	1650

TUNA An oily fish, tuna is a good source of vitamin D and omega-3 fatty acids. Sushi and sashimi are a delicious, low-fat way to consume very fresh fish.

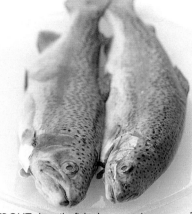

SEAFOOD – FRESH FISH

Nutritionists recommend eating at least two portions of fish, one of which should be an oily fish, each week. Fish is an excellent, low-fat source of vitamins, minerals and protein. Oily fish, such as salmon and mackerel, also contain omega 3 fatty acids, which may help to reduce the risk of arteries clotting.

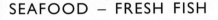

TROUT An oily fish that contains omega-3 fatty acids. It is delicious baked or cooked under the grill.

RECIPE For a low-fat supper, marinate a tuna steak in ginger, lime juice, honey and a little soy sauce for 30 minutes. Chargrill, then serve with steamed rice and stir-fried vegetables.

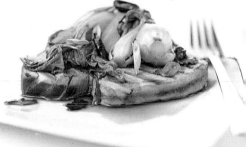

SNAPPER A white fish that is low in fat and high in vitamin B. It has a subtle flavour and is a good fish to use for steaming, baking or grilling.

SALMON A well-known oily fish high in omega-3 fatty acids and protein. Salmon is delicious simply poached or baked and served with lemon or dill.

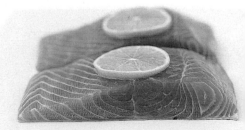

FOOD	CARB	FIBRE	FAT	ENERGY	
	g	g	g	kcal	kJ

SEAFOOD CONT.

FOOD	CARB	FIBRE	FAT	kcal	kJ
groper, 100g	0	0	1	86	360
gumard, 100g	0	0	2	86	390
haddock, smoked, 1 small fillet, 85g	0	0	1	8	35
herring, canned, drained, 125g	10	0	22.5	315	1325
jewfish (mulloway), steamed,					
1 fillet, 145g	0	0	4	128	540
kamaboko, 100g	0	0	1	52	220
kingfish, 100g	0	0	3	105	440
leatherjacket, 100g	0	0	2	93	390
lemon sole, 1 small fillet, 85g	0	0	2	79	330
ling, 100g	0	0	2	93	390
lobster, boiled, 165g	0	0	1.5	159	670
lumpfish roe, 10g	0	0	1	12	50
mackerel, 100g	0	0	16	221	930
mullet, steamed, 1 fillet, 74g	0	0	3.5	99	415
mussels, 100g	0	0	2	87	365
mullet, steamed, 1 fillet, 74g	0	0	3.5	99	415
mussels, 100g	0	0	2	87	365
mussels, smoked, canned in oil, drained, 100g	4.5	0	10.5	193	810
ocean perch, 1 fillet, 120g	0	0	2.5	112	470
octopus, 100g	0	0	1	69	290
oysters, raw, 10, 60g	0.5	0	2.5	72	305
oysters, smoked, canned in oil, drained, 10, 60g	0.5	0	7	124	520
parrot fish, 100g	0	0	2	93	390
perch, 100g	0	0	1	86	360
pike, 100g	0	0	1	88	370
pilchards, 150g	0	0	3.5	157	660
pilchards, canned in tomato sauce, 225g	2	+	29	430	1805
prawn cutlets, fried, 3, 75g	15	+	12	218	915
prawns, garlic, 100g	2.5	+	7.5	121	510
prawns, king, cooked, 100g	0	0	1	104	435
prawns, school, steamed, 150g	0	0	1.5	114	480
redfish, 100g	0	0	2	93	390
salmon, canned in brine, drained, 100g	0	0	9.5	171	720
salmon, patty mix, 100g	0	0	7.5	202	850
salmon, pink, canned in brine, drained, 100g	0	0	6.5	146	615
salmon, raw, 100g	0	0	12	181	760
salmon, red, canned in brine, drained, 100g	0	0	12	194	815
salmon, roe, 1tbsp, 10g	0	0	1	12	50
salmon, smoked, 50g	0	0	2.5	67	280
sardines, fresh, 100g	0	0	2	67	280
sardines, canned in oil, drained, 100g	0	0	15.5	226	950
sardines, canned in tomato sauce, 100g	1	Tr	13	190	800
scallops, steamed, 160g	1	0	2.5	168	705
scampi, 100g	0	0	2	107	450
scampi, crumbed, fried, 2, 100g	0	1	17.5	314	1320
sea bream, 100g	0	0	5.5	138	580

SELENIUM Shellfish contain the trace mineral selenium, a powerful antioxidant that may protect against disease, and have anti-ageing properties.

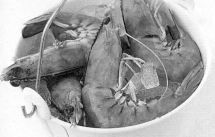

SEAFOOD – SHELLFISH

Although high in nutrients, shellfish also have a reputation for being high in cholesterol. However, cholesterol is present in all animals, and though some shellfish can have a high level, the fact that they are so low in fat, (on average less than 2%), means that they are one of the healthiest forms of protein.

RECIPE For a low-fat dinner, marinate peeled raw prawns in garlic, lime juice, macadamia oil and pepper. Grill and serve with a low-fat yoghurt and diced watermelon dressing.

OYSTERS Their reputed aphrodisiac quality can be attributed to the fact that oysters have the highest zinc content of any food, a mineral needed for growth and sexual development.

VITAMIN B
Shellfish are full of Vitamin B_{12}, which is vital for the growth of new cells and tissues and for the function of the nervous system.

FOOD	CARB	FIBRE	FAT	ENERGY	
	g	g	g	kcal	kJ
SEAFOOD CONT.					
sea perch, 100g	0	0	1	86	360
sea trout, 100g	0	0	2	93	390
shark, 100g	0	0	1	100	420
snapper, steamed, 100g	0	0	2.5	121	510
sole, 100g	0	0	1	81	340
squid, boiled, steamed, 100g	0	0	1	79	330
squid rings, fried, 125g	8.5	0	12	257	1080
trout, coral, grilled, 100g	0	0	2	93	390
trout, rainbow, steamed, 100g	0	0	6	155	650
trout, smoked, 100g	0	0	5	136	570
tuna, canned in brine/water,					
drained, 190g	0	0	5	234	985
tuna, canned in oil, drained, 250g	0	0	28	450	1890
tuna, steamed, 100g	0	0	3	119	500
whiting, all varieties, 100g	0	0	1	93	390
SEAWEED					
raw, average all types, 10g	Tr	1.2	0	1	4
SEEDS					
poppy, 1tbsp	2	+	4	46	195
pumpkin, 50g	5	2.6	7	155	650
sesame, 1tbsp	0	0.8	7	76	320
sunflower, 1tbsp	0.5	0.9	8	88	370
SEMOLINA cooked, 1 bowl, 245g	15.5	+	0	75	315
SHALLOT 25g	N	0.3	0	6	25
SNACK FOOD (see also CORN CHIPS)					
bacon rings, 1 packet, 25g	N	0	6.5	124	520
burger rings,1 packet, 50g	0	1	13	249	1045
cheese & bacon balls, 1 packet, 50g	N	N	17	265	1115
cheese twists, 1 packet, 50g	30	0.5	13	249	1045
cheese potato puff type, 1 packet, 50g	30	0.5	15	258	1085
popcorn, microwave, 1 pack, 100g	4	1	2	32	135
potato crisps, plain, 1 large packet, 50g	25	2.6	15	249	1045
potato crisps, 1 large packet, 50g	N	2.6	16	250	1050
potato crisps, lite, 1 packet, 50g	30	3	15	258	1085
potato crisps,					
average all flavours, 50g	N	2.6	18	282	1185
potato twists, plain, 1 packet, 50g	N	1.3	17	258	1085
pork rind, crackling, 1 packet, 30g	N	0.1	8.5	145	610
prawn crackers, 5, 30g	N	0	2	45	190
pretzels-type, 10g	6.5	+	0.5	37	155
sesame seed bar, 1, 45g	20	+	12	167	700
SNAIL cooked, 2, 30g	N	0	0.5	29	120
SOFT DRINKS – CARBONATED					
(see also CORDIAl, SPORTS DRINKS AND WATER)					
cola, 375ml	39	0	0	150	630
diet cola, 375ml	1	0	0	1	5
dry ginger ale, 375ml	28	0	0	124	520

SOFT DRINKS These tend to be high in sugar and low in nutrients, and should therefore not be consumed on a regular basis. Their high sugar content also means high consumption can lead to dental caries. Small bottles of mineral water are equally easy to carry around, as are 'diet' soft drinks – although these do contain artificial sweeteners such as saccharin.

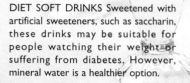

DIET SOFT DRINKS Sweetened with artificial sweeteners, such as saccharin, these drinks may be suitable for people watching their weight or suffering from diabetes. However, mineral water is a healthier option.

COLA With 8–10 teaspoons of sugar per can, these drinks are high in calories. Cola also contains significant quantities of caffeine.

FLAVOURED MINERAL WATER These usually have fruit juice added. They can have a comparable sugar content to a glass of cola or lemonade.

MINERAL WATER The bottles offer a portable alternative to soda water for quenching your thirst. Plain soda waters and mineral waters are free of calories.

RECIPE Combine pineapple juice, chilled camomile tea and soda water to make a delicious fruit-based soft drink.

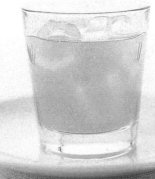

FOOD	CARB	FIBRE	FAT	ENERGY	
	g	g	g	kcal	kJ
SOFT DRINKS – CARBONATED CONT.					
dry ginger ale, diet, 375ml	1	0	0	4	15
orangeade, 275ml	48	0	0	194	815
orangeade, diet, 375ml	1	0	0	2	10
lemonade, 375ml	40	0	0	159	670
lemonade, diet, 375ml	1	0	0	4	15
pineapple & grapefruit flavoured, 375ml	45	0	0	161	675
diet, 375ml	1	0	0	6	25
lemon & lime flavoured, 375ml	40	0	0	179	750
lime flavoured, 375ml	40	0	0	150	630
diet, 375ml	1	0	0	4	15
tonic water, 250ml	0	0	0	82	345
SORBET lemon, 50g	7	0	0	62	260
SOUP					
chicken, low calorie, 220ml	8	N	1	50	210
condensed, beef broth, 220ml	12.5	N	2.5	81	340
condensed, creamy chicken, 220ml	12	N	6	120	505
condensed, creamy chicken & corn, 220ml	14.5	N	7	131	550
condensed, creamy chicken & mushroom, 220ml	15	N	0	70	295
condensed, creamy chicken & vegetable, natural, 215ml	10.5	N	8	139	585
condensed, creamy mushroom, 1 serving, 215ml	7	N	8	139	585
condensed, pumpkin, 1 serving, 215ml	13	N	4	96	403
condensed, creamy minestrone, 1 serving, 215ml	15	N	0.5	74	310
condensed, creamy potato & leek, 215ml	12	N	13	180	755
condensed, minestrone, 220ml	15	+	0	70	295
condensed, mushroom, 220ml	13	N	6.5	126	530
condensed, pea & ham, 220ml	15	+	0.5	94	395
condensed, tomato, 1 serving, 220ml	12	+	0.5	57	240
instant, chicken noodle, lite, 1 mug, 200ml	5	N	0.5	29	120
instant, chicken & vegetable, 1 mug, 200ml	14	N	0	60	250
instant, chunky chicken, 1 serving, 1 mug, 250ml,	31	N	3	167	700
instant, creamy cauliflower & cheese, 1 mug, lite, 200ml	9	N	1	45	190
instant, mushroom & chives, 1 mug, lite, 200ml	5.5	N	1.5	38	160
instant, pea & ham supreme, 1 mug, lite, 200ml	9.5	N	1	55	230
instant pumpkin & vegetable, 1 mug, lite, 200ml	9	N	0.5	40	170
minestrone, reduced calorie, 220ml	10	+	0	50	210
tomato, reduced calorie, 220ml	11	1.5	0	50	210
vegetable, reduced calorie, 220ml	9	1.5	0.5	48	200
SPAGHETTI (see also PASTA)					
canned, bolognaise, 130g	12.5	1.3	0.5	68	285
canned, tomato sauce, 130g	16.5	1	1.3	87	365
canned, tomato sauce & cheese, 130g	16.5	+	1	82	345
SPICES average all types, 1 tsp	0	N	0	9	40

SPICES Just like herbs, spices are used in such small quantities that they usually add little nutritional value to our diet. However, adding flavourful and fragrant spices to your food can allow you to use a lighter hand with the salt and cooking oil. Spices have also been renowned for their medicinal properties for centuries.

GINGER May help digestion, and when chewed or made into tea, can be a good relief for morning sickness.

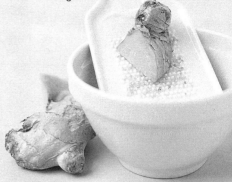

CHILLIS A spicy meal can make the eyes water and the nose run – a good way to bring relief from the blocked airways of a heavy cold.

GARLIC This contains a compound called alliin, thought to help reduce blood cholesterol levels. Its pungent taste and smell make it a great flavouring to add to low-fat dishes.

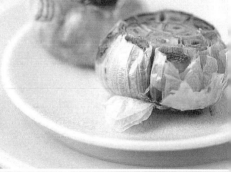

SWEET SPICE Cinnamon, star anise and cardamom are spices that can be used to add flavour to sweet dishes. Infuse in milk, or in a syrup, to poach fruit.

RECIPE For low-fat spicy prawns, marinate peeled and deveined raw prawns in grated ginger, crushed garlic, a finely chopped red chilli and lime juice. Thread onto skewers and barbecue or grill.

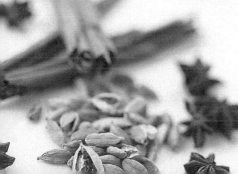

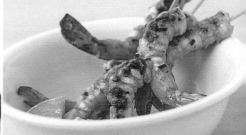

FOOD	CARB	FIBRE	FAT	ENERGY	
	g	g	g	kcal	kJ
SPINACH					
cooked, 35g	0.3	0.7	0	7	28
frozen, cooked, 35g	0.2	0.7	0	7	28
raw, 35g	0.5	0.7	0	9	37
SPORTS DRINKS					
isotonic type, 500ml	36	0	0	150	630
isotonic type, lite, 500ml	N	0	0	144	605
glucose type, 300ml	58	0	0	151	635
glucose type, lite, 500ml	N	0	0	100	420
SPREADS (see also HONEY AND JAM)					
almond spread, 100g	19	+	54	571	2400
cheddar cheese, 1tbsp	0	0	5	60	250
cheddar cheese, light, 1tbsp	1.5	0	3.5	48	200
gherkin, 1tbsp	9.5	+	0	57	240
lemon-flavoured, 1tbsp	13	0	1	59	250
marmalade, orange, 1tbsp	9	0	0	34	145
nut and chocolate, 1tbsp	N	0	6	105	440
peanut butter, crunchy, 1tbsp	3.5	1.2	10.5	125	525
peanut butter, crunchy lite, 1tbsp	6	+	7.5	112	470
peanut butter, smooth, 1tbsp	2.6	1	10.5	125	525
peanut butter, smooth lite, 1tbsp	6	+	7.5	112	470
pickles, low-calorie, 1tbsp	N	0	0	8	35
sandwich spread, 1tbsp	6	0.2	2.5	47	195
vegemite, 1tsp	0.5	0	0	8	35
yeast extract, 1tsp	Tr	0	0	8	35
SPRING ONION raw, 12g	0.5	0	0	2	10
SPROUTS					
alfalfa seeds, sprouted, raw, 100g	4	+	0.5	29	120
lentils, sprouted, raw, 100g	22	+	0.5	106	445
mung beans, sprouted, raw, 100g	4	1.5	0.5	31	131
radish seeds, sprouted, raw, 100g	3.5	+	2.5	43	180
soya beans, sprouted, raw, 100g	9.5	+	6.5	121	510
wheat seeds, sprouted, raw, 100g	42.5	+	1.5	198	830
SQUASH					
acorn, baked, 70g	9	2.2	0	39	165
buttemut, baked, 70g	5	1	0	22	94
STAR FRUIT (CARAMBOLA)					
raw, 100g	7.3	1.3	0	32	136
STOCK CUBES all varieties, 1, 5g	1	0	0,5	11	45
STOCK POWDER all varieties, 1tbsp	2	0	0.5	19	80
STRAWBERRIES					
canned in syrup, 100g	17	0.7	0	65	279
raw, 100g	6	1.1	0	27	113
STUFFING average, small serving, 30g	6.5	0.5	2.5	56	235
SUET MIX 100g	10	0	90	807	3390

ISOTONIC This means that the drink contains the same concentration of carbohydrates as blood, so the carbohydrates can be easily absorbed and blood sugar levels topped up.

SUGAR Sports drinks do not generally contain less sugar than other soft drinks. In fact, they are often high in calories and sugars.

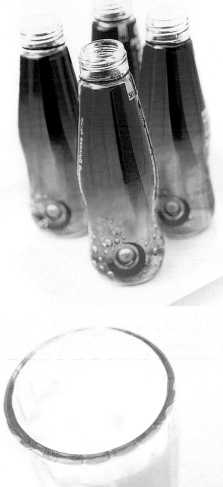

SPORTS DRINKS Many people

believe sports drinks are more 'healthy' than other soft drinks, yet they do contain a lot of sugars such as dextrose and glucose syrup, which are high in calories. Many of the drinks provide mineral salts, which are lost through sweating, but only highly trained athletes are likely to need this additional source.

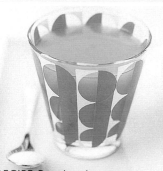

RECIPE People who engage in a lot of exercise could mix orange juice with water and a tiny amount of salt and sugar as a healthy alternative.

SODIUM Sports drinks have added sodium to speed up fluid absorption. Salt lost through perspiration can be replaced through food or even a glass of milk.

FOOD	CARB	FIBRE	FAT	ENERGY	
	g	g	g	kcal	kJ
SUGAR					
average, 1 tsp	5	0	0	19	80
any type, 1 tbsp	17	0	0	64	270
icing, 1 tbsp	20	0	0	76	320
SULTANAS dried, 1 tbsp	13.5	0.5	0	55	230
SUSHI					
Californian roll, 5 pieces	N	N	2	139	585
inari (bean curd pouch with rice), 85g	N	N	2	130	545
nigiri, 30g	N	N	0.5	30	125
SWEDE					
peeled, boiled, 150g	3	1	0	16	69
SWEET POTATO					
peeled, boiled, 100g	20.5	2.3	0	84	358
raw, 1, 235g	50	5.6	0	56	237
SWEETS (see also CHOCOLATE)					
boiled, 1	5	0	0	15	65
butterscotch, 1	5.5	0	0	24	100
caramels, 1	4	0	0	24	100
fruit gums, 30g	27	0	0	8	35
fudge, 2 pieces, 35g	28.5	0	4.5	155	650
jaffas, 55g	N	0	18	245	1030
jelly babies, 1	3.5	0	0	15	65
jellybeans, 1	3	0	0	11	45
liquorice allsorts, 100g	77	2	5.2	349	1483
liquorice pieces, 100g	65	1.9	1.4	278	1185
peppermints, 1 packet	N	0	0	84	355
marshmallows, 1 packet, 85g	68	0	0	283	1190
sesame seed bar, 45g	N	+	12	167	700
sherbet lemons, 1	N	0	0	20	85
toffees, 1	3.5	0	0.5	20	85
SWISS CHARD raw, 30g	1	N	0	6	25
TACO					
with meat & bean sauce,					
1 serving, 180g	N	+	14	231	970
TAHINI paste, 1 tbsp	0.2	1.6	11.8	121	510
TAMARILLO (TREE TOMATO)					
raw, peeled, 90g	4	+	0	24	100
TANGERINE raw, peeled, 100g	8	1.3	0	35	147
TAPIOCA cooked, 1 bowl, 265g	18.5	0.3	0	75	315
TEA					
for each teaspoon of sugar in tea, add ...	5	0	0	19	80
black, no sugar, 1 cup, 250 ml	Tr	0	0	Tr	Tr
with whole milk, 1 cup, 250ml	1	0	1	18	75
with skim milk, 1 cup, 250ml	1.5	0	0	13	55
TINNED FRUITS (see also FRUIT SALAD)					
peach & mango in syrup, 133g	12	1	0	56	235
sliced peaches in syrup, 133g	18	1.2	0	71	300
fruit salad in syrup, 125g	15	1.5	0	59	250

TOFU

Made from soya beans, these are low in fat, high in calcium and excellent sources of protein for vegetarians. All soya products contain phytoestrogens, which are hormone-like substances in plants. Although opinion is divided, some studies suggest that these substances may help to protect women from breast cancer and symptoms of the menopause.

FIRM TOFU This holds its shape well when cooked. It can be marinated and then fried or grilled, or cut into pieces and added to curries. Store in water in the refrigerator.

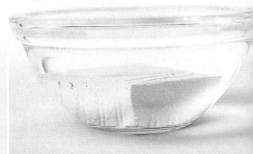

SILKEN TOFU This soft tofu can be blended and used instead of dairy products in dips, ice creams or cheesecakes. It is also wonderful as a simple dessert sweetened with bananas and maple syrup.

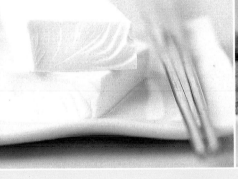

TEMPEH A fermented soya bean cake, this Indonesian food has a nutty taste and can be thinly sliced and grilled, or used in stir-fries.

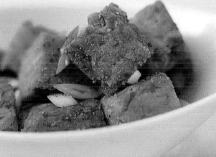

RECIPE Marinate thick slices of firm tofu in a mixture of grated ginger and soy sauce for several hours. Fry, grill or add to a stir-fry.

FOOD	CARB	FIBRE	FAT	ENERGY	
	g	g	g	kcal	kJ
VEAL CONT.					
leg steak, untrimmed, fried, 1, 100g	0	0	4	159	670
liver, grilled, 85g	1.5	0	7	159	670
loin chop, lean, baked or grilled, 1, 50g	0	0	1.5	73	305
loin chop, untrimmed, baked or grilled, 1, 55g	0	0	2.5	88	370
schnitzel, fried, 1, 85g	8.5	N	23	287	1205
shank, lean, simmered, 1, 80g	0	0	2	117	490
shank, untrimmed, simmered, 1, 90g	0	0	6	160	670
shoulder steak, lean, grilled, 1 small, 50g	0	0	1.5	73	305
shoulder steak, untrimmed, grilled, 1 small, 55g	0	0	2.5	84	355
VEGETABLE JUICE, average, 250ml	11	0	0.5	51	215
VEGETABLES (see INDIVIDUAL VEGETABLES)					
VENISON roast, 100g	0	0	5.5	157	660
VINEGAR					
apple cider, 100ml	6	0	0	14	60
unspecified, 100ml	15.5	0	0	21	90
white, 1tbsp	0	0	0	4	15
WAFFLES					
frozen, 1 square, 35g	13.5	1	2.5	88	370
homemade, 1 round, 75g	24.5	2	10.5	218	915
WATER (see also SOFT DRNKS)					
plain mineral, soda, tap, 1 glass, 250g	0	0	0	0	0
bottled, average, all varieties, 1 glass, 250g	0	0	0	0	0
WATER CHESTNUTS					
canned, drained, 40g	3.5	+	0.5	19	80
raw, 5, 50g	12	+	0	49	205
WATERCRESS raw, 32g	0.5	0.5	0	6	25
WHEATGERM 1tbsp	1.5	0.8	0.5	17	70
YAM baked or boiled 100g	37.5	1.7	0.4	153	651
YEAST					
dried, bakers, compressed, 1 sachet, 7g	0.5	N	0	8	35
dried, brewers, 1 sachet, 7g	0.5	N	0.5	19	80
YOGHURT					
acidophilus, live, low-fat, 100ml	11	0	0	56	235
acidophilus, plain, 100ml	8	0	3.3	24	100
bio type, acidophilus, low-fat, honey & strawberry, 100ml	13	0	3	100	420
black cherry, with live cultures, 100ml	17	0	4	104	435
drinking, apricot, 250ml	31	N	5	190	800
drinking, 100ml	13	0	1	81	340
drinking, swiss type, vanilla, 250ml	31.5	N	5	184	775
drinking, vitamin-enriched, 250ml	24	N	5	139	585
drinking, fruit, 250ml	31.8	N	5	190	800
frozen, fruit, 100ml	20	0	5	132	555
frozen, fruit yoghurt stick, raspberry, strawberry, 85ml	20	0	5	132	555
frozen, low-fat, 100ml	N	0	3	114	480
frozen, low-fat, flavoured, 100ml	22	0	0	83	350

VEGETABLES Try to eat at least five portions of vegetables and fruit each day. Vegetables are high in fibre and are packed with vitamins and minerals. Choose from fresh, frozen, raw and canned varieties, but bear In mind that vegetables lose vitamin C if stored for a long time or are cooked for too long in a lot of water.

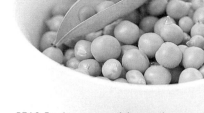

PEAS Fresh peas are delicious, but are not always available. Frozen peas are convenient and a good source of vitamins and fibre.

BROCCOLI A rich source of vitamin C and folic acid, broccoli is also associated with antioxidant properties.

CORN An excellent source of vitamin C, a good source of fibre and a moderate source of thiamin and niacin.

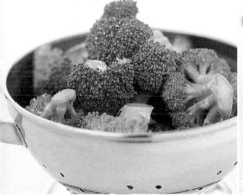

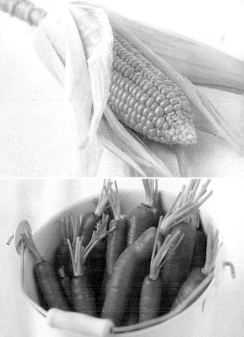

RECIPE To prepare vegetables without adding fat, steam some vegetables, drizzle with lemon juice and sprinkle with black pepper.

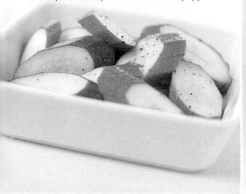

CARROTS Rich in betacarotene, an antioxidant that may help prevent chronic diseases such as heart disease. Carrots are the best source as there is no evidence that betacarotene supplements have any benefit.

FOOD	CARB	FIBRE	FAT	ENERGY	
	g	g	g	kcal	kJ
YOGHURT CONT.					
frozen, low-fat, low sugar, 1 cone	N	0	0	45	190
frozen, fat-free, honey, 1 cone	N	0	0	109	460
frozen, reduced-fat honey, 1 cone	N	0	0	90	380
frozen, strawberry, 85ml	N	0	4	127	535
fruit cocktail, diet lite, 100ml	13	0	0.2	92	385
honey, dairy style, 100ml	11.5	0	7	132	555
kiwifruit & mango, diet lite, 100ml	13.6	0	0.2	94	395
lemon, cultured, 100ml	15	0	0	82	345
low-fat, berry, diet lite, 100ml	15	0	1	87	365
low-fat, berry fruits, live, diet lite, 100ml	7	0	0	43	180
low-fat, fruit salad, blueberry, cherry,					
diet lite, bio type, 100ml	7	0	0	43	180
low-fat, passionfruit, 100ml	16	0	0	89	375
low-fat peach, diet lite, bio type, 100ml	6.5	0	0	42	175
low-fat, peach & mango, diet lite, 100ml	15	0	2	194	815
low-fat, plain. dairy type, 100ml	6	0	0	51	215
low-fat, strawberry, diet lite,					
bio type, 100ml	6.5	0	0	42	175
low-fat, summer fruits, diet lite, 100ml	16	0	1	93	390
low-fat, vanilla, diet lite, bio type, 100ml	6	0	0	40	170
low-fat, vanilla, fruit & nut, diet lite,					
100ml	16	0	1	40	170
plain, bio type, 100ml	5	0	4.5	95	400
plain, dairy type, 100ml	6	0	8	120	505
plain, skim milk natural, 100ml	7	0	0.1	51	215
plain, swiss style, creamy custard, 100ml	1	0	4.5	107	450
plain, traditional, dairy type, 100ml	6.5	0	35	77	325
soft serve, 100ml	16.5	0	0	80	335
soft serve, low-fat, average	N	0	0	80	335
soft serve, natural, 100ml	24	0	2	142	595
soft serve, fat-free, 100ml	4.5	0	0	21	90
strawberry delight, 125ml	20	0	4	136	570
vanilla, cultured, 100ml	19	0	4	114	480
yoghurt, cultured, 65ml	11	0	0	46	195
yoghurt, baby type, banana/vanilla, 100ml	N	0	4	107	450
yogurt, average, all flavours, 150ml	N	0	5	167	700
YORKSHIRE PUDDING					
small serve, 50g	12.3	0.5	5	104	437
ZUCCHINI					
green, boiled, 90g	1.5	1	0.5	13	55
yellow, boiled, 90g	1	1	0.5	17	70